Fashion Journalism

Fashion Journalism

History, Theory, and Practice

Sanda Miller and Peter McNeil

Bloomsbury Academic
An imprint of Bloomsbury Publishing Plc

B L O O M S B U R Y
LONDON · OXFORD · NEW YORK · NEW DELHI · SYDNEY

Bloomsbury Academic

An imprint of Bloomsbury Publishing Plc

50 Bedford Square	1385 Broadway
London	New York
WC1B 3DP	NY 10018
UK	USA

www.bloomsbury.com

BLOOMSBURY and the Diana logo are trademarks of Bloomsbury Publishing Plc

First published 2018

ISBN: HB: 978-1-4725-2017-3
PB: 978-1-4725-3581-8
ePub: 978-1-4742-6966-7
ePDF: 978-1-4742-6965-0

Library of Congress Cataloging-in-Publication Data
Names: Miller, Sanda, author. | McNeil, Peter, 1966- author.
Title: Fashion journalism : history, theory, and practice / Sanda Miller and Peter McNeil.
Description: London, UK ; New York, NY, USA : Bloomsbury Academic, an imprint of
Bloomsbury Publishing Plc., 2017. | Includes bibliographical references and index.
Identifiers: LCCN 2017043803 | ISBN 9781472520173 (hardback : alk. paper)
Subjects: LCSH: Fashion writing.
Classification: LCC TT503.5 .M55 2017 | DDC 808.06/674692—dc23 LC record available at
https://lccn.loc.gov/2017043803

Cover design: Liron Gilenberg
Cover image: DIOR: AUTUMN/WINTER 2000/2001 PRET A PORTER
(© THIERRY ORBAN/Sygma/Getty Images)

Typeset by Integra Software Services Pvt. Ltd.
Printed and bound in India

To find out more about our authors and books visit www.bloomsbury.com.
Here you will find extracts, author interviews, details of forthcoming events and
the option to sign up for our newsletters.

CONTENTS

LIST OF FIGURES

PREFACE

In *Fashion Journalism: History, Theory, and Practice,* writing and ideas come together. It is the companion to *Fashion Writing and Criticism*, a historical and theoretical work on fashion criticism published by its authors in 2014. *Fashion Journalism: History, Theory, and Practice* takes advantage of both academics' roles as writers who at times have also worked for the popular press, particularly Miller's forty-year career in the print media as well as broadcasting. Miller has taught university students this topic for many years, and now shares her distinctive approach to writing for and about fashion.

It is almost a cliché from undergraduate to Ph.D. candidates that many people are anxious about writing. Our aims and objectives are firstly to provide a didactic manual that encourages fashion, art, design, and other such students to write without fear. More importantly, a new dimension is added—we work together with students in order to learn how to find inspiration for both writing and styling beyond the world of "Google," useful as Google might be; indeed, everyone now uses it for reference and information. Full of exciting examples from the great traditions of humanistic art, literature, music, philosophy, and also the beauty of the everyday, *Fashion Journalism: History, Theory, and Practice* empowers students to access the visual richness that is required of the fashion designer as much as the fashion writer.

There is a growing awareness around the world that there is a general crisis concerning ignorance of the "culture of fashion," even among those who work in the industry. A design manager for *Hermès* will have problems working for the company if they do not understand the role of equitation (horse-riding) in the early modern period and the appearance of the *Amazone* (the well-dressed female horse-rider in the nineteenth century, represented in the art of Edouard Manet, for example).[1] Taking an instagram shot and finding the most beneficial and interesting hashtags involve an understanding of light, color, and composition, as well as word play and allusion. The "culture of fashion" is more than a scaffold in a design, critical, or styling career. It is central to generating and understanding

---

[1] We thank our French friends at Diktats Bookstore, Nicolas and Antoine, for discussing the state of fashion education today.

new ideas. As the sociologist Sally Weller notes, fashion is a "complex, multi-dimensional form of knowledge" as well as being a technology of garment mass production (Weller, 2007: 39). If fashion is a form of knowledge, then the profession requires you to develop many types of knowledge, including the visual. Finding visual inspiration outside your immediate field is also therefore a concern of this book.

The work aims to teach you how to look for yourself rather than word-searching, simply sitting at home and browsing the web or reproducing the millions of (sometimes banal) photo-stock images that are all around us. How do you bring an expanded sense of the world around you into your fashion orbit? How do you rise to the top and leave the ordinary behind? Is there a way to go beyond the few words relevant on instagram?

We address the student directly on these points. Everything a student of fashion journalism needs is contained in this book. *Fashion Journalism: History, Theory, and Practice* explains the established categories in journalism. Students learn that writing is not a collection of ideas laid down on paper but necessarily carries a structure. The six "famous questions"—*what, who, why, where, when, how?*—the latter being the key point in journalism—are applied to fashion writing, in order to demystify writing and to demonstrate that writing *can be learned*. Through a series of case studies and examples drawn from everything from art to current affairs, students learn the structure and logic required to create a piece of succinct writing. Whether fashion writing is the same as news reporting in cognate areas is a key topic tackled throughout this book.

ACKNOWLEDGMENTS

The authors wish to thank the anonymous reviewers at Bloomsbury and our editors Ariadne Godwin and Frances Arnold, as well as Pari Thomson, for their patience.

Sanda would like to thank the two most important people in her journalistic career, both of whom gave her support and enabled her to become a journalist (albeit on a freelance basis).

The first presence was the maverick and magnificent literary editor of *The Times*, the late Philip Howard (1933–2014), whom Wikipedia introduced as "the distinguished journalist who worked for over 50 years for *The Times* … (educated at Eton and graduated with a First Class Degree in Classics at Trinity College, Oxford)." Philip gave Sanda the chance to review a book for him. The year was 1984 and she continued to review for him on a regular basis until he decided to give up his literary editor's role in 1993.

The second presence was the distinguished BBC 3 radio producer Piers Plowright (gently referred to as a radio legend), with whom she collaborated between 1984 and 1998 (when Piers Plowright retired) researching and compiling documentaries ranging from art and philosophy to cookery.

She would also like to thank her colleagues and friends at Southampton Solent University, where she is Research Fellow (after working there for seventeen years as Senior Lecturer), and her wonderful colleagues at the fashion college *Istituto Marangoni*, London. It was for the Marangoni students that she returned to journalism in order to create a unit to teach students how to write for the press. This unit was the starting point for Peter and Sanda's book. Finally, Sanda would like to thank her family— Noa, Giulia, and Neil—for being family!

Peter would particularly like to thank the participants in "Fashioning the Early Modern," an EU-funded project led by Evelyn Welch which ran from 2010 to 2013, especially John Styles, who generously shared his wide knowledge regarding the history of print and eighteenth-century newspapers. The discovery of certain images in this book and their related photography was made possible while Peter was a Fellow at the Lewis Walpole Library, Yale University. He is also grateful to Aalto University for appointing him Distinguished Professor within the FiDiPro "Costume Methodologies" project (2014-2018) funded by the Academy of Finland, allowing him to work more closely with European colleagues, including his coauthor. He wishes to thank Professor Sofia Pantouvaki and the many other collegiate researchers within the 'Costume

Methodologies'/ Academy of Finland major funded project as well as the Aalto University Costume in Focus (CiF) research group. Friends and colleagues who assisted with details of the manuscript and picture research include Kristen McDonald of the Lewis Walpole Library and Virginia Wright, Launceston. He also thanks Bathurst Regional Art Gallery for a residency at the bucolic Murray's Cottage in Hill End, New South Wales, at which he was able to consider final stages of this manuscript. The Centre for Contemporary Design Practices in the Faculty of Design, Architecture and Building at UTS also supported the project. Finally, he thanks his graduate students past and present, particularly Masafumi Monden, and wishes Anthony O'Brien returned health.

This book is dedicated to the friendship of Sanda and Peter, who were brought together by historical and contemporary research about fashion.

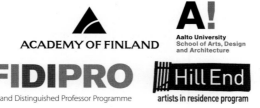

With support by the "Costume Methodologies" research project of Aalto University within the Finland Distinguished Professor (FiDiPro) scheme

1

Introduction—Fashion Journalism: Fun—Not Frightening

Unlike the notion of "fashion criticism," which still raises some eyebrows regarding its ontological status (does it even exist?—and in some sense it clearly does, as we are discussing it here, even if not in the sense in which the reader of our book might have anticipated)—fashion journalism is all around us. We read and hear reports about fashion both past and present in the press, on the television, at the movies, and online on our computers and handheld devices—from iPads to mobile phones. Can we therefore talk about "fashion journalism" as an independent category of journalism? The answer is yes, and it is much easier too than in the case of "fashion criticism," because within the modern practice of journalism we are inundated with a multitude of newly created categories of journalism, and even if some are oxymora, many appear to be functioning well. Moreover, a growing number of contributions on the subject address this very issue, such as Julie Bradford's recent book *Fashion Journalism* (Routledge, 2015).

Our book will be concerned with print journalism, for example, writing for newspapers and magazines, and the two questions we set out to answer are: (a) can we count "fashion journalism" among the latter? (b) if so, in what way does "fashion journalism" differ from journalism generally, and if this be indeed the case, in what way does it make a contribution to journalism?

Among the specialized categories of journalism which include such popular subjects as sports, science, and investigative journalism, we can perhaps add a splendidly idiosyncratic category—*gonzo*—because we believe that it may reflect the practices of a vast number of journalists, especially those who write about fashion, calling themselves "fashion journalists" instead of acknowledging (of course, that would never do!) that what they practice is *gonzo* journalism. Invented in 1970 by journalist Hunter

S. Thompson (1937–2005), *gonzo* journalism is defined by Wikipedia as "a style of journalism without claims to objectivity, which disregards the rigours of newspaper journalism and replaces it with a personal approach, whereby sarcasm, humour, exaggeration and profanity are the order of the day." Is it an adequate category to be predicated of "fashion journalism?" Our assumption is legitimate enough given that unlike other specialized types of journalism, "fashion journalism" appears at times to function on the principles associated with *gonzo* journalism. We shall return to this issue later.

By analogy with the specialized categories of journalism listed above, "fashion journalism" can also be defined as a specialized category dealing with fashion in all its ramifications to include key aspects such as the commercial and business aspect (the business of the fashion industry—indeed "BOF" is the name of a much-read Web site), which is what the majority of people assume fashion is all about. This is certainly not the case—fashion is not just about commerce—and we find confirmation if we glance at the list of contents in Bradford's book that incorporates the latest developments in the area. Some of the key issues she selected are working in fashion journalism, fashion media, the fashion industry, ideas, sources and interviewing, writing fashion news and features, reporting the catwalk, reporting the trends, styling, photography and video for online, fashion blogging and social media, and finally fashion journalism and PR (Bradford, 2015). It is immediately obvious that we can distinguish two main areas of inquiry: theoretical (writing and reporting on fashion) and the fashion industry itself, with some interesting additions such as "styling."

Why, then, are we still faced with so much disdain when the word "fashion" is mentioned in the same breath as journalism? The reason is simple: on the one hand, the fashion industry is a multi-million dollar, pounds, or EURO enterprise which contributes significantly to the GDP of a country (that is good!); on the other hand, it has succeeded over many centuries to create for itself the reputation of being frivolous, disengaged from reality, and catering for the privileged few—not something that good Marxists, many Feminists, and Ecologists approve of in a hurry (that is bad!) and yet and yet this apparent conflict has created a new criticality around the topic (a good thing!).

Our book will be divided into two parts: Part One "Understanding Print Journalism," presents the long history of the practice and the development of the "news" introducing at the same time those who created it: the journalists, as a new profession Part Two "Understanding Fashion Journalism," addresses fashion journalism as a specialized category of journalism that arose within it, and it is divided into three chapters: History, Theory, and Practice. Chapter 6 in turn is subdivided into four sections, each introducing one key category of fashion journalism: hard news (we question its validity in fashion journalism), the feature, the interview and profile and the review.

We hope that by the end of our journey we will have established a link between the general principles of journalism and how they apply to "fashion journalism" and also to have determined the nature of the original contribution of fashion journalism as a self-sufficient category of journalism.

Aims and objectives

The following questions will be addressed in this book:

- What is journalism and how can we apply established categories of writing to the fashion world?
- How do we write a professional "copy" for the press?
- How do we structure a range of categories both in print and fashion journalism, such as "features," the interview, the profile, the review (the work of the art critic), and the report (the work of the fashion reporter we may also call, as in the case of the likes of Suzy Menkes, the fashion critic).
- What are the sources of inspiration that take journalism in general and fashion journalism in particular beyond the **merely factual in the first instance and the merely descriptive in the second?**
- How is the visual imagination required in fashion writing to be developed and improved?
- Are recent developments in media (the web, the blog, the noncommercial press) producing new forms of writing, or are they in part also based on the professional standards applied in journalism?

We start with the question "what do students need in the 'age of google?'"—both in terms of theory and practice. The answer is to study both the theory and practice of fashion journalism as part of the wider category of journalism, where it belongs:

a. **Theory:** Students will learn that writing is not a stream-of-consciousness-like technique whereby you write down whatever passes through your mind; on the contrary, writing for the press requires rigorous structuring, and to start with, students will have to memorize the six "famous" questions used in journalism that are to be asked when structuring a piece of writing—**why? where? when? who? what? how?**—and successfully apply them in fashion journalism (it should be noted that such concepts can be applied to structure many other forms of writing, from the abstract ([summary of a work] to a presentation of research findings).

b. **Practice:** Through a series of case studies drawn from the press, students will learn two things: (a) how the professionals "do it" and (b) through practice, for example, reading and reading more, the students will learn to become critics themselves by assessing "who is doing a good job?" and "why are they good at it?"

Thus, students will learn that good journalistic practice need not be difficult, mystical, or frightening, but should be fun! This book will enable students to develop their creative and writing abilities in order to produce exciting and informative articles fit for the new century.

Each of the three relevant terms used in the title of the book—(a) journalism; (b) theory; (c) practice—will be defined and explained: we will start by defining the profession of the journalist over time, after which we introduce the main types (categories) of journalism used at present in print media.

Next we move to theory, and we find out that some of the theoretical frameworks have been purloined from other disciplines and put to good use in journalism.

Then we will move to practice, and this section will function in a manner analogous to that of the "snapshots" introduced in our previous book *Fashion Writing and Criticism,* enabling us to demonstrate the practice of writing journalism with examples from the national press and specialized magazines. The aim is to demonstrate "how it is done" (the practical work of the journalist), and some examples will address the important issue of learning to analyze and form judgments.

We will explore the traditional categories of journalism such as the *feature*, the *interview*, the *profile*, and *criticism*. These are all terms employed by fashion journalists, but we intend also to critically assess the usefulness of such "appropriations" in theory (is it useful, necessary, or even illuminating to employ "deconstruction" in fashion writing—a strategy borrowed from philosophy used in architecture, for example?) and how (or does it?) work in practice. This will enable us to further explore whether interviewing somebody working in the fashion industry or writing a profile of a fashion designer need be in any way different from any other interview. Here comes the oxymoron—because the answer is (of necessity)—yes. But what actually happens is that we do not need to produce a separate type of interview/profile; in fact, the opposite is the case—the well-established categories of journalism we got on to list are applicable to the world of fashion, and to prove this, we chose as our case study a profile of Tom Ford. The framework is the same but the subject matter differs, so that in our example (a "profile") only the interviewee differs and so does the subject matter, but nothing else is altered.

The list of contents for the book is as follows:

Part One, Chapter 2 considers the history of print journalism. We start with a historical trajectory of print journalism from the seventeenth-century

English news-books or "corantos" (Price, 1998: 418) to contemporary multimedia. We pass through the six principal categories (types) of journalism. These include:

> *Hard News*: Facts are relayed straight. This deals with facts, events, and information—the most "objective" form of journalism.
>
> A special category of hard news is *investigative news*, which aims to uncover the truth about a particular subject, person, or event. A well-publicized case was that of Rupert Murdoch, the Australian-born media mogul and owner of *The Sunday Times*, *The Sun*, and *The News of the World*. Following allegations of phone-hacking practices at *The News of the World*, which was investigated by Lord Levenson (*The Levenson Enquiry*) and which took place on the April 25, 2012, in London, Rupert Murdoch denied all knowledge of such practices at his newspapers, but in the end he was forced to close *The News of the World*.
>
> *Feature writing*: We move away from the objective approach of the news writer to the subjective approach of the feature writer. Essentially, a feature can be defined as a topical story seen through the lenses of its author. David Randall in his seminal book entitled *The Universal Journalist* (Pluto Press, 2011) suggests that there are fifteen distinct categories of feature writing, which will be listed below, but from his list we place under different headings the interview, the profile, and the review.
>
> (i) **color piece**: describing a scene and throwing light on its themes
>
> (ii) **fly on the wall**: reporting the goings-on as a fly on the wall might see them; this style is more efficiently used in television documentaries. One of the famous early examples of such a technique was the 1975 cult film now hailed in part as a "fashion film," *Grey Gardens* by the Maysle Brothers, Albert and David. The Brothers used an unobtrusive handheld camera to track the eccentric but loving relationship between two faded and reclusive society figures (a mother and daughter) who were direct relatives of Jackie Kennedy. One year of film footage—which included occasional questions and interjections from the filmmakers—was edited into about 1.5 hours. This was the derivation of *Big Brother* and other such reality TV shows, although an artificial environment has to be created in order to engender the isolation of the behavior in the latter. The idea that truth is often stranger than fiction is at the basis of many such films.
>
> (iii) **behind the scenes**: this style is similar to fly on the wall but the journalist is incorporated as part of the event

(iv) **in disguise:** pretending to be another person

 (v) **the interview:** this is one of the categories of writing which will be separated from feature writing and treated independently.

(vi) **the profile:** as with the interview we single out the profile for "special" treatment and we will take the magnificent "Lunch with the FT" (*Financial Times*, UK) (weekly profiles of the most important people in the world of politics, business, culture, arts, and sport) as our template.

(vii) **how to:** this type of article assists readers by explaining how to do something and the writer may learn about the topic through research, interviews with experts, or personal experience.

(viii) **fact box/chronology:** a simple list of facts, perhaps in chronological order

 (ix) **backgrounder:** a history of an extended fact box

  (x) **full texts:** extracts from books or transcripts of interviews

 (xi) **my testimony:** a first-person report of an event

(xii) **analysis:** an examination of the reasons behind an event

(xiii) **vox pop/expert roundup:** a selection of views from members of the public

(xiv) **opinion poll:** survey of public opinion

 (xv) **the review:** the job of the critic. As in the case of the interview (number v) and the profile (number vi) we will single out the job of the reviewer (critic) which formed part of the subject of our previous book, *Fashion Writing and Criticism*, for separate analysis. At this point we must emphasize that criticism and journalism are not the same thing, hence the need for this new work.

The Interview. Technically, an interview is a dialogue rather than a conversation, the only difference being their final aim, in the former instance summed up as an exchange while in the latter the relationship is altered whereby the interviewer is also the questioner whose aim is to uncover something about the interviewee.

The profile. For some reason, the profile is given short shrift by book authors and the reason might be that this particular category sits in between interviewing and the feature; no wonder David Randall considers it as a feature and this is what he says: "Normally a study of a personality at the centre of a story, but it can be also the portrait of a place, organisation, religion, etc. It can be a report of one encounter with the subject, or gather many views and give a rounded portrait" (Randall, 2011: 220–3).

The Review. What is a review? A good question, but the answer is
more complicated than it appears *prima facie,* and this may well have
something to do with words. In journalism the job of the critic comes
under the label of "reviewer," which can cause confusion and we
often found ourselves in the position of having to explain to people
that the "reviewer" is in fact the "critic." The situation is further
complicated by the fact that in fashion journalism we do not have
reviews but reports—the fashion journalist "reports from" rather than
"reviews" the fashion show, although for the last three decades we
also have "fashion reviewing" because we have fashion exhibitions
in art museums that add a layer of complexity and difference to the
field. Such a situation would have been however unimaginable before
Diana Vreeland changed that by conferring upon Yves Saint Laurent
the status of artist, that is, she organized a "retrospective"—as if he
were a Claude Monet or other great artist—at the Costume Institute
of the *Metropolitan Museum of Art,* New York (1983–4), and her
brave (also brazen?) gesture opened the door to a "newish" category
for the fashion writer: reviewing fashion exhibitions.

In fact, Miller is proud to have pioneered this kind of reviewing for the
established magazine *Apollo.* In 2004, she approached its editor Michael
Hall with a proposal—if she could review for the magazine the exhibition
entitled "'*Shocking*': The art and fashion of Elsa Schiaparelli," which after
being shown in Philadelphia arrived at the Musée de la mode et du textile
in Paris (September 2003–January 2004). With the word "art" in its title
combined with the fact that Schiaparelli regarded herself (to Gabrielle
Chanel's disdain) an artist, rather than a fashion designer and had close
links with the Surrealists, the editor agreed and so the first review of a
fashion exhibition in a British art magazine was published (*Apollo,* August
2004). Three years later, in the July/August 2007 issue, its editor Michael
Hall started his editorial as follows:

People sometimes express surprise that *Apollo* publishes reviews of
exhibitions on fashion. Even scholars of what used to be called "the
decorative arts"—which now seems to want to be known as "material
culture"—can be surprisingly dismissive of a subject that is often
perceived as frivolous and ephemeral. I have always found it hard to
understand why anybody who cares about visual things should dismiss
fashion, as it is the one art form, apart of course from architecture, that
is inescapable, unless you choose to spend your life in a naturist camp. In
any case, the history of fashion is now a lively academic discipline with
a great deal to say about the relationship of fashion to the other arts.
This is especially evident in the *V&A* "Surreal Things" exhibition, which
explores a trail long since blazed by such scholars as Richard Martin, in
his book *Fashion and Surrealism,* published 20 years ago. (p. 15)

Chapter 3 "A New Profession: The Journalist"—here we provide an historical overview of being a journalist, and in spite of the reputation (some) journalists acquired of being uneducated hacks, we want to show that we are in fact dealing with a venerable profession. If we are to consider the maverick Pietro Aretino to be the "father" of journalism (see Chapter 2), then journalism is a profession with a long pedigree, also featuring in later periods many women as participants.

In this chapter we return to the eighteenth century and the "inauguration" of the professional journalist, which is less impressive than it sounds because it simply means "pay me for my work"!

In Part Two, Chapter 4 "Fashion Journalism: History" traces the long backstory that led toward the dedicated fashion periodical, including consideration of the rise of print, the seventeenth-century journal *Mercure galant*, and the proliferation of journals throughout the nineteenth century. From the 1890s the cost of paper and printing dropped dramatically in price and as the burgeoning middle classes felt an obligation to read about and form opinions on topics as different as the art in their emerging public galleries and what women were wearing to go shopping in the new department stores, journalism flourished. "Penny" papers and other very cheap formats provided news on a myriad of topics for all classes of society. We feature some charming and also some cutting images here that indicate that "anxiety" attended the fact that working women were engaging with fashion news. They also point to the paradox that at precisely the time women were demanding suffrage and better working conditions they were more likely and able to engage with novel dress fashions, a source of concern to some reformers.

Chapter 5 "Fashion Journalism: Theory" concerns the theoretical framework of journalism, and yes—it has its theory. Two key books need to be referenced at this point, both dealing with the variety of theories which have been appropriated by the new academic discipline "Fashion Studies" in order to create a theory of its own. Whether it works, it is necessary, sufficient, or even relevant; that is another matter, but the study of fashion at university level still enjoys a certain novelty. Two useful books that can be consulted here, both published in the same year, are:

(a) Malcolm Barnard (ed.), *Fashion Theory: A Reader*. Routledge Student Readers, 2007

(b) Linda Welters and Abby Lillethun (eds), *The Fashion Reader*. Berg, 2007

Chapter 6 "Fashion Journalism: Practice:" asks: who are the fashion journalists? What is their combination of academic background, practical skills, good networking abilities, talent for writing, or is it maybe the *gonzo* approach of the charismatic "celeb" that makes the difference today? In order to unpack this section we have selected the following categories of mainstream journalism adopted and most widely used in fashion journalism: "The feature" "The interview and profile" and "The critical review". When Sanda Miller started to write for *The Times* in 1984, its "celeb. lit.ed." (literary editor) Philip Howard taught her all that there was to know about journalism: firstly, "do not write long sentences because the little old lady from Neasden [a small English town] by the time she manages to reach its end would have forgotten the beginning," and secondly, "crack a joke or two, dear girl" (i.e., humor always helps)—and so, bearing in mind these important pieces of advice, Miller became a journalist following her training as an art historian, writing for Howard to start with. It was at that point that her real apprenticeship began, and she realized that writing for the press was not a piece of cake either. Both Miller and McNeil respect the role of the editor, and always hope for a good one! Prose often has to be modified, and this can be at odds with how college students and academics feel about their "freedom."

The two authors will therefore concentrate on the following categories of journalism relevant to *fashion* journalism: feature writing, the interview, the profile, and the review. But we provided also a section on "fashion news" with a question mark attached to it: is there such a thing as fashion journalism? Or is this *gonzo* journalism? The conclusion we reached is that news and fashion do not make good bedfellows!

This section will be based on case studies from the press and specialized magazines: we will select high-profile ("celeb") interviews or profiles from a high-quality publication (such as *The Financial Times*, *Vogue*, *Vanity Fair*) and analyze them in order to show how professional journalists approach the subject. This practice will enable students to not only learn the "tools" of the trade but also to become aware of the qualitative differences between a good and a mediocre—miserable even—piece of writing, thus becoming the critics themselves in the process. In an age when anyone can set word to keyboard or mouse or smartphone or other device and comment on many aspects of news—indeed, the comments sections of digital news almost insists upon leaving a response—how can that response go beyond either simply opinion, or abuse, or anger and make a real contribution?

PART ONE

Understanding Print Journalism

2

The History of Print Journalism—From Written to Printed Media

The origins of the "media" as a system of communication

The intriguing and splendidly alliterative subtitle of Roger Parry's book *The Ascent of Media: From Gilgamesh to Google via Gutenberg* evokes notions of grand venerability for the media, by tracing it back to the Assyro-Babylonian hero "Gilgamesh," whose identity was based on that of the king of Uruk, who reigned between 2800 and 2500 BCE (Guirand and Schmidt, 2006: 91). Thus the ascent of "media" can be traced back to prehistoric times—defined in the most basic way as communication—and in that sense, Parry argues, the first cave paintings from 38000 BCE years can be thus defined.[1] He suggests seven steps of communication, starting with its graphic manifestation (Drawings/Paintings/Signs), the oral (Sermons/Speeches/Theatre), the written (Scrolls/Letters/Posters), the printed (Books/Newspapers/Magazines), the aural (Radio/Telephone/Recording), the visual (Film/TV/Photography), and the digital (Web/Multimedia).

Given this wide use of the word "media," how can we even hope to provide a definition, for as Parry observed:

> Put "media" into Google and you get more than one billion results. It's a very broad term. The search reveals that Media was an ancient region of Asia near the Caspian Sea that flourished about 1,000 years before the

---

[1] In her recent, pathbreaking book on the history of costume (Bloomsbury 2017), Donatella Barbieri argues that the Lascaux cave paintings also represent the first representation of costume for performance.

fall of Rome. It is roughly where the Kurds live today. That is the first recorded use of the word, but is only relevant to this story in that the region happens to be the source of what is now the English language. (Parry, 2011: 7)

Apart from providing the first known example of the use of the word, albeit as a proper name, Parry provides an analysis of the term, as well as reproduces the *Oxford English Dictionary* definition of the word:

> The word "medium" is both an adjective and a noun. As an adjective it means average, with alternatives being "intermediate" and "middle." As a noun it is defined as "means," with the alternatives of "vehicle," "channel," and "mode." It is the use of medium as a noun that is the subject of this book. It is the vehicle by which words, images, information, and ideas are distributed. Content is *mediated* if it reaches us through the agency of a *medium*.

The *Oxford English Dictionary* defines media as "the main means of mass communication (esp. newspapers and broadcasting)." The American *Webster's* goes for "any means, agency or instrumentality of communication." The more contemporary *Encarta* has "the various means of mass communication thought of as a whole, including television, radio, magazines and newspapers" (Parry, 2011: 7).

Parry distinguishes sixteen main channels or vehicles used to convey the "four basic elements of speech, music, images and writing" that he regards as the basic tools developed over millennia by humans for communication purposes, which include "books, newspapers, television and so on" (Parry, 2011: 8).

Leo Tolstoy: The expression theory of art

Parry's statement that communication happens through speech, music, images, and writing finds unexpected support from a less well-known source: the Russian writer Leo Tolstoy, who wrote in 1897 an essay entitled *What Is Art*, in which he introduces an "expression theory of art," whereby the work of art becomes the vehicle which transmits. Tolstoy actually uses the words "transmitting" and "receiving," anticipating the communication theories that emerged during the twentieth century based on the system of transmitter/receiver, two terms first used by Claude Elwood Shannon in his book *A Mathematical Model of Communication* published in 1948. By this, Tolstoy means the act of artistic creation as embodied in the work of art when transmitted to their rightful receiver, the public. A communication theory is proposed here with Tolstoy's example, "speech" being one of A. Parry's four channels of communication:

Every work of art causes the receiver to enter into a certain kind of relationship both with him who produced, or is producing, the art, and with all those who, simultaneously, previously, or subsequently receive the same artistic impression.

Speech, transmitting the thoughts and experiences of men. (Tolstoy in Feagin and Maynard, 1997: 169)

Tolstoy proposes that a work of art is a vehicle which mediates between transmitter (the artist) and receiver (the public), but what is being transmitted is not a vacuous aesthetic experience (he was no adherent of Charles Baudelaire's "art for art's sake" theory), because for Tolstoy the process of artistic creation amounts to a great deal more, namely that of embodying the artist's emotions that are conveyed to the public through his art. This theory is known in aesthetics as the "expression theory of art" and it emerged during the Romantic period, of which Tolstoy—alongside philosophers such as Benedetto Croce, R. G. Collingwood, and Suzanne Langer—is the main proponent. Tolstoy defined it thus:

Art is a human experience consisting in this, that one man consciously, by means of certain external signs, hands on to others feelings he has lived through, and that other people are infected by these feelings and also experience them. (Tolstoy in Feagin and Maynard, 1997: 171)

While music and images are valiant and exciting means of communication, what is relevant in this context is the written word, itself a development from oral communication that included "speech."

The "written" and the "printed" media

At this point an important distinction needs to be introduced between the **written** and the **printed** word, the former traced back by Parry even before Gilgamesh, to about 5500 BCE when a member of an extinct civilization the Harappan – and these examples are the earliest known – pressed or made marks in ceramics, later succeeded by the earlier known form of writing:

We think, but do not know as we cannot read them, that the symbols indicated the contents of the pot. These fragments are the earliest-known surviving examples of writing. Some 4,000 years later we know that a scribe called Sin-lique-unninni made a copy of the oral legend of King Gilgamesh on clay tablets in a language called Sumerian using a writing technique called cuneiform. He is cited as the world's first-named author of a story and subsequent scholarship means that we are able to read what he wrote. (Parry, 2011: 17)

Mesopotamia (Greek for "between two rivers") created the first large urban settlements or towns, irrigation to manage erratic rainfall and grow crops, and a system to trade their cereals for the minerals and woods they did not themselves possess. By marking clay with a sharp tool, they created writing: "that incomparable process for transpiring, we might say, thoughts and feelings, for materializing them, fixing then outside of a person like so many independent and concrete objects, and thus communicating them to others, everywhere, in time and space" (Jean Bottéro, 2004: 8–9). This writing system was fully in place by 3200 BCE. If we leave out the "oral," "aural," and "visual" aspects of the media, with regard to the written word, the span between the written and the printed work takes us from 3500 BCE to the Middle Ages and 1450, when the printing press was invented in Germany by Johannes Guttenberg (1398–1468), with the next *volte face* emerging during the twentieth century. Its importance was famously summed-up by the Canadian writer Marshall McLuhan in his book entitled *Understanding Media: the Extensions of Man*, first published in 1964 through the dictum "The medium is the message" regarded by now the slogan which sums up what media studies are all about.

Marshall McLuhan: The medium is the message, but what does it mean?

What is less well known is the unexpected context in which these words appear in McLuhan's erudite book. He takes his cue from the eighteenth-century British empirical philosopher David Hume (1711–1776), whose repudiation of causality continues to make philosophers scratch their heads. Hume proposed that cause and effect are not connected but merely conjoined; they simply follow each other rather than being linked by an *a priori* (not observable by experience) causation chain.

In 1739–40 when Hume was merely twenty-eight years of age, he published the *Treatise of Human Nature*, whose total lack of success was famously summed by Hume himself later in his autobiography entitled *My Own Life* (1776), in which he stated:

> Never literary Attempt was more unfortunate than my Treatise of human Nature. It fell dead-born from the Press; without reaching such distinction as even to excite a Murmur among the Zealots. (Mossner in Hume, *Treatise*, 1969: 17)

Little wonder, because this is where we find not one but two definitions of causation:

> A CAUSE is "an object precedent and contiguous to another, and where all the objects resembling the former are plac'd in like relations of

precedency and contiguity to those objects, that resemble the latter." If this definition be seen defective, because drawn from objects foreign to the cause, we may substitute this other definition in its place, viz: "A CAUSE is an object precedent and contiguous to another and so united with it, that the idea of the one determines the mind to form the idea of the other, and the impression of the one to form a more lively idea of the other." (Hume, *Treatise*, 1969: 220)

McLuhan quotes Hume in relation to the process of mechanization:

Mechanization is achieved by fragmentation of any process and by putting the fragmented parts in a series. Yet, as David Hume showed in the eighteenth century, there is no principle of causality in a mere sequence. **That one thing follows another counts for nothing. Nothing follows from following, except change.** (McLuhan in Marris and Thornham, 1999: 40)

What follows is even more unexpected, because the explanation of "the medium is the message" hinges on one of the main principles: that of **simultaneity** on which Cubism is based, whereby the three-dimensional object is broken down (**faceted**) and re-organized on the flat surface of the canvas, and so the "fourth dimension" of time is eliminated. McLuhan quotes from E. H. Gombrich's book *Art and Illusion,* where the latter introduced Cubism as "the most radical attempt to stamp out ambiguity and to enforce one reading of the picture—that of a man-made construction, a coloured canvas" (McLuhan in Marris and Thornham, 1999: 41). Based on Gombrich, McLuhan provides his own explanation of Cubism, on which he deduces the famous words "the medium is the message":

For cubism substitutes all facets of an object simultaneously for the "point of view" or facet of perspective illusion ... In other words, cubism, by giving the inside and outside, the top, bottom, back, and front and the rest, in two dimensions, drops the illusion of perspective in favour of instant sensory awareness of the whole. Cubism, by seizing on instant total awareness, suddenly announced that *the medium is the message.* (McLuhan in Marris and Thornham, 1999: 41)

While it is perfectly true that the Cubists cared little about narrative or subject matter (content), focusing exclusively on its formal complexities which presupposed the faceting processes mentioned by Gombrich, this process of faceting was only completely eliminated by the even more radical versions of cubism such as *Orphism* and later *Purism,* which are self-referential, e.g., contentless, so the form becomes the content. This is exactly the point made by McLuhan. From Cubism he expands into other fields of inquiry, including media, and then in a charmingly rhetorical manner he uses the argument from analogy to prove that the same principles are applicable elsewhere, communication included:

> Specialized segments of attention have shifted to total field, and we can now say, "The medium is the message" quite naturally. The message, it seemed, was the "content," as people used to ask what a painting was *about*. Yet they never thought to ask what a melody was about, nor what a house or dress was about. In such matters, people retained some sense of the whole pattern, of form and function as unity. But in the electric age this integral idea of structure and configuration has become … prevalent. (McLuhan in Marris and Thornham, 1999: 41)

McLuhan is not totally right about music, because it can be argued that just like storytelling, music does not only have form but also content: Beethoven's *Sixth Symphony* ("The Pastoral") is explicitly programmatic in content, so the relationship form/content is analogous to what we have in the visual arts. With dress, however, we must introduce a third term, "function," which replaces "content," e.g., the form of dress is dependent on what it is for: protection, adornment, conceptual investigation, etc.—and whether we can further argue that function is the same as content or not is a matter of semantics, so we have permutations of the three terms here: **form, content, function.**

McLuhan lists "dress" alongside architecture, long established as a form of visual arts: The form of a garment is dependent on what it is for, e.g. its function: skirt, shirt, cape, doublet … and not the other way round so that we can re-phrase "the medium is the message" to "the medium is determined by the function." We are left, however, with an important field: communication. How does it work in this instance to say that "the medium is the message": if we look at the list of media which evolved over the millennia as listed by Parry, we find a similar situation—the medium (the scroll, the poster, the book, the newspaper) does indeed determine the message, each to their own, we could say! But we want a complete overlap where message and media are coextensive and we can find it in the digital era of web and multimedia. It is at this point that McLuhan's "the medium is the message" is re-visited and, given that he postulated it in the 1960s, becomes prophetic:

> In the 1960's Canadian writer Marshall McLuhan described media as the extensions of man and talked of the creation of a global village. With the arrival of the internet and the web, his predictions have come true. (Parry, 2011: 3)

And it is indeed the digital era that implemented McLuhan's prediction: "the medium is the message," as Parry observed:

With the arrival of the internet and the web, his predictions have come true. "We have been hit hard by seismic shifts wrought by the web ... Media is profoundly being transformed," said Steve Forbes, publisher of *Forbes* magazine, in a memo to his staff in 2009. This emphasizes the magnitude of the economic challenge posed by converting content into digital code. (Parry, 2011: 3)

From the "written" to the "printed" media: The invention of the printing press

We associate the invention of the printing press with fifteenth-century Germany and the name of Johannes Gutenberg, but printing, defined as "the process of reproducing an image from an original," originated in China around 800 AD. This process was different from Gutenberg's press in as much as the Chinese used wooden blocks with which they reproduced both texts and images (Parry, 2011). The pioneers of the modern printing technique associated with Europe, however, were Gutenberg (1398–1468) in Germany, William Caxton (1422–1492) in England, and Aldo Manutio (1449–1515) in Italy, who Latinized his name to Aldus Manutius, but Gutenberg is credited with the invention of printing.

Gutenberg had been the manufacturer of pilgrims' mirrors a decade before his printing début. In 1454, Gutenberg exhibited at the Frankfurt Fair the trial pages of his masterpiece, a Bible, that he would go on to produce in 180 identical copies. Europe's book-owning classes were not slow to understand the importance of what this man had achieved. Attempts to protect the secret of the new technology were unavailing. Soon craftsmen were introducing the new technique of book manufacture to all corners of Europe (Pettegree, 2014: 58–9) (Figure 2.1).

English merchant William Caxton, contemporary with Gutenberg, lived first in Bruges, where, after a sojourn in Cologne, he set up a press in 1472, publishing his first English text in 1473. In 1476, he moved to England and set up the first press in that country; his first published book there being was Geoffrey Chaucer's *The Canterbury Tales*. But the honor of publishing the first bible in English fell to another person: the scholar William Tyndale (1494–1536), who paid dearly with his own life for the privilege at a time when bibles were still written in Latin rather than vernacular. He was executed, but the Tyndale Bible became a ground-breaking book on which the King James Bible published in 1611, still used to-date, is based.

The third printer of note is the Venetian Aldus Manutius who started his printing press in 1495 with an edition of Aristotle, followed by other

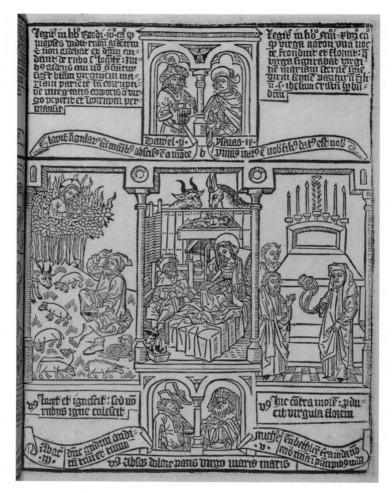

FIGURE 2.1 *"Biblia Pauperum" (Pauper's bible), block-book possibly printed in Holland, possibly in a British binding, printed c1465, woodcut on paper in morocco leather binding, blind stamped. Bought under the terms of the Murray Bequest, Victoria and Albert Museum E.687–1918. © Victoria and Albert Museum, London.*
   The page is carved from a single wood-block, inked, and then printed, and shows Old and New Testament scenes. This type of printing preceded books made with movable type (invented c1450) and continued to be produced after the latter as they were cheaper.

Greek classics such as Aristophanes, Sophocles, and Thucydides. Inspired by ancient Roman coins, he adopted for his press an imprint of a dolphin wrapped around an anchor to which the motto *Festina lente* (hasten slowly) was added. What was even more remarkable was that these printing establishments provided—in a way similar to eighteenth-century coffee houses—centers for discussion. Historian John Hale notes that they were full of noise and life, with "resident scholarly staffs," illustrators, and translators (Hale, 1994: 288). Aldus was particularly annoyed not only because of the multitude of letters "of learned men" which "would cost him whole days and nights if I were to reply" but above all by the multitude of visitors to his shop who slowed him down:

> Then there are the visitors who come, partly to greet me, partly to see what new work is in hand, but mostly because they have nothing better to do. "All right," they say, "let's drop in on Aldus!" ... I say nothing of those who come to recite a poem to me or a piece of prose, usually rough and unpolished, which they want me to publish for them. (Hale, 1994: 288)

But book publishers only covered part of the needs for communication: they were either printing the ancient classics which survived in manuscript form, or they were printing the work of established contemporary writers, or they published the bible, and these books were expensive and exclusive. That is the reason why an important need related to communication was not able to attract the attention of the pioneering printers and publishers: the news!

A radical invention: News in print!

It is in the nature of human beings to be curious: curious about each other, curious about what goes on around them, curious about what is happening in the world they live in, and the way this curiosity was satisfied in the past was often through word of mouth. That could be achieved in a variety of ways, not least by using a messenger, which carried its own risks embodied in the "don't shoot the messenger" dictum whose origins are nebulous, but which is meant to convey a simple idea, namely not to take revenge on the bringer of bad tidings.

In the Middle Ages the marketplace or the main square in the town was a hub where information exchange across Europe happened and a lot more besides, including entertainment even of the grim sort, such as executions. Medieval market towns were "about 30 miles apart" and made the long-distance travel that characterized the burgeoning trade and prosperity of Western Europe possible (Pettegree, 2014: 118).

The cathedral or church, too, was an important space for sharing news and gossip and even for making graffiti and very material acts of poetry (*posy*), which is common in English medieval churches. Fleming argues that writing was much more fluid than we think of today, and done on parchment, jewels, textiles, ceramics, and walls (Juliet Fleming: *Graffiti and the Writing Arts of Early Modern England*, 2001). Unlike today, churchgoers moved around and were very noisy, and the church generally faced the square anyway, so there was sure to be something going on. Shopping and trading were frequently done after Mass, and church was not the somber affair that we think it is today.

Another important hub for news exchange were the drinking establishments: the tavern and the inn where people gathered to eat and drink, womanize, and exchange information. Taverns go back to the Romans, where there were as many as one every thirty feet in the town of Pompeii. People ate simple food a bit like tapas there, drank a great deal, and discussed a range of topics from what is the best time of day to make love, to what type of God did the Jews worship (the drinkers were all men of course, apart from the courtesans). We find this ambiance in a letter written by one of the most famous Venetians, who can justly claim the honor of being the first journalist:

The first journalist: Pietro Aretino

Pietro Aretino's (1492–1556) prolific writing activities included quantities of letters from which he himself selected 3,000 for publication in book format, which were published by his friend, the printer Francesco Marcolini. Apart from the letters, his prolific output included the *Raggionamenti: The Erotic Lives of Nuns, Wives and Courtesans* published in two volumes in 1534 and 1535 respectively. He was also the author of the notorious *Sonetti lussuriosi* (*Lust Sonnets*), written to accompany Giulio Romano's erotic drawings engraved by Marcantonio Raimondi, and the even more notorious *I Modi* (*The Ways*) or *The Sixteen Pleasures,* the latter attracting to him the label of pornographer.

For this reason history punished him, because after his death his name disappeared from records, although never completely, until the twentieth century when he was resurrected by none other than avant-garde poet Guillaume Apollinaire. Apollinaire published his own lugubrious piece of pornography, *The Eleven Thousand Virgins* (*Les onze mille Vierges*), which Picasso himself regarded as a masterpiece. A few years before World War I, Guillaume Apollinaire published two new editions of the cobbler's son (Aretino): he edited a new version of the *Ragionamenti* he found, very likely by accident, in the Bibliothèque des Curieux and compiled an anthology of Aretino's writings for a series which Rémy de Gourmont directed for the *Mercure de France.* Slowly Aretino took his place (in France to start with but then in other countries, including his native Italy) beside Boccaccio, the *Célestine* of Rojas and the Restoration playwrights of England (Stafford: Introduction in Aretino, 1971: 14).

Considering both his prolific output and versatility, it is only right to confer on Aretino the accolade of the *first journalist*. In the introduction to a volume of selected letters, its translator, the eminent Renaissance scholar George Bull, wrote:

His (Aretino's) literary versatility was extraordinary ... [T]hey range over art and politics, war, sport and religion, and city life or country pleasures of every sort. This diversity of subject-matter has helped to characterize Aretino as the first journalist. He made his money and reputation by the high-speed production, for a wide, educated public, of letters or broadsheets that may be seen as the Renaissance equivalent of the leaders, features, art criticism, gossip columns and eye-witness reporting of modern times. (Bull: Introduction in: Aretino, 1976: 13)

A perfect example of his satirical style which earned him the accolade of "Scourge of the Princes" is a lengthy letter entitled "A Dream of Parnassus" addressed to Signor Gian Iacopo Lionardi, dated 6 December 1537. In it Aretino recounts a nightmarish dream, worthy of Dante's "Inferno," in which he finds himself at the foot of mountain Parnassus and he sees how from above "slither masses of men, screaming so hideously that it is a cruel and outlandish joke to see them snatching at shrubs and stumps, sweating and shitting blood." The devilish vision is subsequently replaced by an inn, which was Aretino's next port of call:

But there I was in an inn, established for the purpose of mulcting the murderers of poetry. When I was inside, I could not refrain from exclaiming: "As Cappa said, 'Who hasn't been inside a tavern, doesn't know what Paradise is,' and as my stomach found its appetite restored I decided to eat my fill for once." (Aretino, 1976: 139)

So where did taverns fit into everyday life during the Renaissance?

Taverns and the news

Taverns were a ubiquitous part of early modern society. It has been estimated that in England alone there were 20,000 drinking establishments: about one for every twenty adult males in the population (Figure 2.2). It is unlikely continental Europe was any less well served. Aside from the church, with which the tavern coexisted in a relationship of undisguised competition, this was the quintessential gathering place of early modern society. It was a volatile environment in which to share the news (Pettegree, 2014: 129).

Both inns and taverns could include wealthy establishments whose function transcended that of providing mere food and/or accommodation. Thus, during the fourteenth century innkeepers, in addition to providing food and accommodation, played an important role in the provision of banking services for the international merchant community. 'Many money brokers set themselves up as innkeepers, and many innkeepers acted as brokers'. (Pettegree, 2014: 130)

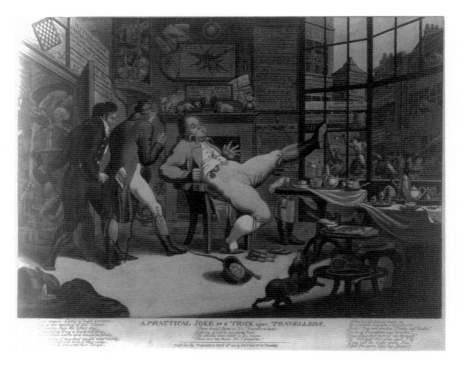

FIGURE 2.2 *"A practical joke or a trick upon travellers": Pubd. for the Proprietors, April 16th, 1810 by S. W. Fores, No. 50 Piccadilly, 1810, aquatint with color. Courtesy Library of Congress Prints and Photographs Division, Washington DC PC 1—11657 (B size) [P&P].*
In this image a "travelling prig" has a joke played upon him when spurs are dropped in one of his boots. He is surrounded by an untidy assortment of coffee, tea, wine, "rich cordials," and spirits; it is breakfast as eggs and honey are being served. A crowd outside the tavern is smashing the windows of a coach under the advertising sign "foreign spirits."

The humble version of the tavern, at the time when Aretino was writing, were "raucous places, full of noise: boisterous, smelly and frequently violent. People came to let off steam, to celebrate with friends, and to forget the cares of a harsh and punishing life" (Pettegree, 2014: 131). But like their grander equivalents, the humble inns and taverns played their part:

> These more humble places were also important hubs of communication. Patrons would discuss the issues of the day, pass on rumours and sing together. It was expected that strangers would join the conversation; the solitary traveller who sat alone was often an object of suspicion, and in many places regulations obliged innkeepers to report the names of strangers who took rooms for the night. Even dingy village taverns provided the opportunity for travelling players and musicians to offer impromptu entertainment. (Pettegree, 2014: 131)

The emergence of the pamphlet and news-book

We can link the earliest forms of news printing to the Reformation, which provided a useful vehicle for the dissemination of printed news. This major cultural event commenced with Martin Luther (1483–1546), a professor of Theology at the University of Wittenberg, who started a campaign against the Catholic church initially at doctrinal level but which evolved into an international revolt causing an irreconcilable split within the church; Luther certainly was a fine academic, but not of the gentle kind:

> He was inordinately rude and bad-tempered. His language was often unrepeatable. Rome, to him, was the seat of sodomy and the Beast of the Apocalypse. (Davies, 1997: 484)

What angered Luther to start with was the appearance in Germany of "indulgences" (a remission against sin issued by the Pope and sold in the streets) sold by a friar, Johann Tetzel, and the consequence was Luther's famous 95 *theses against indulgences* that he nailed on October 31, 1517 (All Saint's Eve) on the door of Wittenberg's castle church (Davies, 1997). This public defiance was considered as "Europe's first mass-media event":

> The quantity of books and pamphlets generated by interest in Luther's teaching was quite phenomenal. It has been estimated that between 1518 and 1526 something approaching eight million copies of religious tract were placed on the market. This was a very one-sided contest. Luther and his supporters were responsible for over 90 per cent of the works generated by the controversy. (Pettegree, 2014: 69)

The Reformation regenerated the ailing book industry with the major commercial European centers such as Venice, Augsburg, and Paris at the fore in the publishing industry.

It was very much due to his friend, the brilliant painter Lucas Cranach the Elder (1472–1553)—who arrived in Wittenberg at the invitation of Frederick III (the Wise), Elector of Saxony—that we have Luther's iconic portrait subsequently disseminated throughout Europe via woodcuts. Luther then became the first European "celeb": "In an age where few outside the ranks of the ruling classes would ever have had their portrait taken, this gave Luther a celebrity status that greatly enhanced his aura" (Pettegree, 2014: 70) (Figure 2.3).

It was also the Cranach workshop which designed the pamphlets (*Flugschriften*)—of small format (about 20 × 8 centimeters) and between eight and twenty pages long, beautifully designed by Lucas Cranach, who created their distinctive appearance: their brand identity:

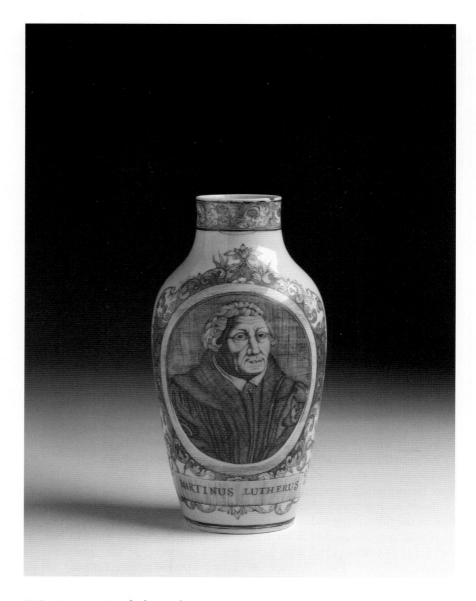

FIGURE 2.3 *Jingdezhen, China, export porcelain vase painted in black enamel with a portrait of theologian Martin Luther, inscribed "Martinus Lutherus"; ca. 1730–60. Basil Ionides bequest. Victoria and Albert Museum C.48–1951. © Victoria and Albert Museum, London.*

Possibly painted after mezzotint prints made in 1714–15 by John Faber the Elder (c.1660–1721), a portrait miniaturist and printmaker born in the Netherlands and subsequently active in London around 1696–8.

Many of Cranach's designs were eye-catchingly beautiful works of art in miniature to honour the words of the man of God. The success of the Reformation pamphlets also helped printers and booksellers appreciate the commercial benefit of brand identity, a significant step towards the development of serial publication. Customers responded by binding the pamphlets together in an impromptu anthology, which is how many have survived today. (Pettegree, 2014: 70)

"Broadsides" is the English word for the one-sided printed sheets that were nailed to church doors, street corners, trees on commons, and other public places, encouraging public reading and viewing. They covered topics such as new laws and controversies and often made use of verse and the sense of the human voice, particularly song.

Invention of the news-book

The publication of such pamphlets intensified with the invention of the "news-book": the *Neue Zeitung* (the current German word for newspaper, but during the sixteenth century its meaning was derived from the Middle German word *zidung*, [the English *tiding*]). The earliest extant *Neue Zeitung* is dated 1509, but after 1530 they became commonplace. The news-books, which were very similar in format to pamphlets, were dedicated to international politics: thus, the 1509 news-book reported the Italian wars, while the 1510 one reported on the "reconciliation of the French king and the Pope."

On the whole, the news-books were "sober and restrained in tone." The title-pages took pains to emphasize that these reports came from authentic sources. Very often the title-pages declared that their text was "received from a trustworthy person" or reproduced a letter sent from abroad "to a good friend in Germany." Sometimes, they reproduced verbatim a despatch written by a captain from the camp or scene of battle. In this way the news pamphlets invoked the trust that reposed in correspondence as a confidential medium between two persons of repute, to bolster the credentials of publications that were now commercial and generally available (Pettegree, 2014: 74–5).

The first forms of newspapers: *Corantos*, manuscript, and printed newssheets

The growing interest in political international affairs created in England a lucrative market to publish such information, initially translated from French and Dutch sources, but this was not well received by the Scottish king James VI (1566–1625), who in 1567 also became king of England as James I, where he ruled until his death. Consequently, the earliest English publications were printed in Amsterdam, which remained a significant site of illicit printing for many centuries until the nineteenth century, printing many French Revolutionary pamphlets and pornographic satires, for example.

> In December 1620, the enterprising Pieter van den Keere published a new periodical entitled the *Courant out of Italy, Germany etc.* This was a straightforward translation of the Dutch edition, published in the same single-sheet format. It was sufficiently successful for van den Keere to maintain publication for the best part of a year. Success brought imitation: by 1621 several of these single-sheet "corantos" were in circulation. The most successful, though prudently attributed to the Amsterdam firm of Broer Jansz, may actually have been printed in London, and from September 1621 the London publisher Nathaniel Butter was openly advertising his responsibility for what was in effect a continuation of van den Keere's series (Pettegree, 2014: 195).

If the "high-brow" corantos can be regarded as the starting point for news journalism, a lighthearted type of publication consisting of "the publication of literature, entertainment and various currents of opinion" which preceded the corantos can be traced back to the sixteenth century. Some of these, such as Simon Fish's "A Supplication for the Beggars" (1529), concerned anti-Roman Catholic opinion, while for other publishers it was more lucrative to write about crime and criminals (Price, 1998: 418–19).

The date of publication of the first newspaper seems to be debatable, mostly for semantic reasons. Thus, Pettegree (2011: 182) credits a book dealer Johann Carolus from Strasbourg who initiated a weekly manuscript newsletter that by this date was common in Europe. By 1605 he acquired a print shop in order to produce a printed version of the manuscript. The earliest surviving copies, which date from 1609, give us an idea of how they looked:

> Individual issues have no title-heading: the title is given only in the printed title-page supplied to subscribers so that they could bind together the year's weekly issue. Instead the news begins, rather like the *avvisi*, at the top of the first page ... a sequence of news reports gathered by their place of origin and dated according to their date of despatch: "From Rome, 27 December," "From Vienna, 31 December and 2 January"; "From Venice, 2 January." The order reflects the sequence in which the posts from these various stations arrived in Strasbourg. (Pettegree, 2014: 183)

Parry provides a different account, while acknowledging the difficulty in finding a common definition for what would constitute the first newspaper:

A *Zeitung* (the German word for news-sheet) was published in what is now the Netherlands in 1609). Copies survive of a 1610 news-sheet from Basle, Switzerland. A number of Dutch printers produced fairly regular *corantos* (meaning currents or flows) with international news useful to shipping companies. (Parry, 2011: 140–1)

Be that as it may, what is certain is that both of the precursors of the modern newspaper belong to the seventeenth century, a period which is often considered to form the bedrock of modernity, rather than the eighteenth, as many people assume (Stone, 1965).

The first "real" newspapers: The Paris and Oxford/London *Gazettes*

On May 30, 1631, the first edition of the Paris *Gazette* was published by Théophraste Baudot, a brilliant doctor who had studied medicine at Montpelier and after returning to his native London met Armand de Richelieu and through him obtained exclusive rights to "print, sell and distribute newspapers within the kingdom" (Pettegree, 2014: 201). England, too, had its own *Gazette* published during the Restoration:

> The first real newspaper in England came after Cromwell had been deposed, when the restored Charles II and his court fled to Oxford in the autumn of 1665 to escape the plague in London. Wanting something to read and fearing that the somewhat unreliable news-sheets coming up from London might be infected with germs, the court authorized the university, which had the technology and skills, to publish the *Oxford Gazette*. (Parry, 2011: 141)

When the court returned to London, so did the *Gazette*, which changed its title accordingly to the *London Gazette*, and it is still with us today. We see it being retailed in the street by a plebeian woman in one of the famous "cries of London," meaning the appearance and sound of street sellers (Figure 2.4). But the *London Gazette* was publishing in troubled times: first, the plague and one year later the Great Fire of London, which the newspaper reported in great detail. This was an important moment in the history of London immortalized by two famous seventeenth-century diarists: Samuel Pepys (1633–1703), whose diaries provide a unique eye witness account of the "Great Fire," and John Evelyn (1620–1706), whose diary, first published in 1818, is an equally important primary source to study life in seventeenth-century London. We can indeed turn to them for information or "color" about the event: "Everybody talking of the dead." Pepys wrote simply of the fire; it made "a noise like the waves of the sea" (Briggs, 1994: 167).

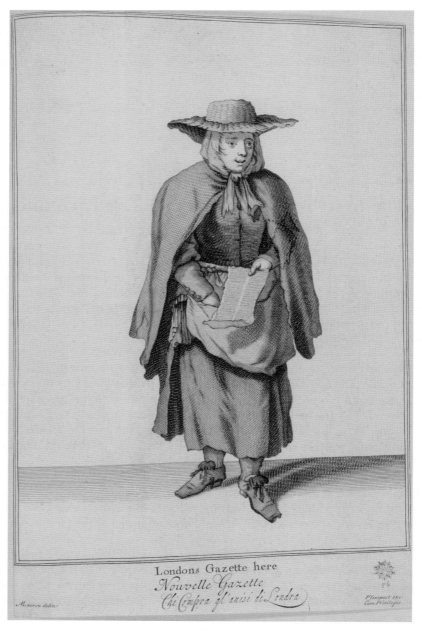

Londons Gazette here
Nouvelle Gazette
Chi Compra gl'auisi di Londra

FIGURE 2.4 *Marcellus Laroon (1653–1702)*, London's Gazette Here/London's Gazette here = Nouvelle Gazette = Chi Compra gl'auisi di Londra, engraving, in The cryes of the city of London: drawne after life in 74 copper plates = Les cris de la ville de Londres: dessignez apres la nature = L'arti com[m]uni che uanno p[er] Londra: fatte dal naturale/P. Tempest excudit. *Courtesy Lewis Walpole Library Yale University, Quarto 75 L328 733.*

Understanding print culture

The coffee house as *locus* for a new phenomenon: The "public sphere"

Peter Borsay's famous account of the English urban Renaissance argued that newspapers were both cause and effect of the development of a new urban culture that was present beyond the London metropolis (Borsay, 1989). Benedict Anderson's ideas of imagined communities strongly argued that "print capitalism [...] made it possible for rapidly growing numbers of people to think about themselves, and to relate themselves to others, in profoundly new ways" (Anderson cit. in Law: 185). Denser urban spaces both demanded and encouraged people to come together. They were the same kinds of spaces that encouraged the rise of fashion, consumption of luxuries, and the development of commercialized leisure—balls, operas, the theatre. The first coffee-shops opened in London in 1652 (Petegree, 2014), and the first advertisement for the new beverage and the new public place created to serve it, creating a whole culture around its drinking rituals dated 1657 published in *The Publick Adviser*: "In Bartholomew Lane on the back side of the Old exchange, the drink called Coffee, which is a wholesome and Physical drink, having many excellent vertues" (Parry, 2011: 33). Coffee and the coffee houses became a worthy replacement of the tavern, where instead of ale, people drank a sophisticated exotic new drink of foreign importation, coffee: "heretofore in use amongst the Arabians and Egyptians" and they spread from Oxford (1650) to London and towns such as Bristol (Briggs, 1994: 168).

In 1989, the German philosopher Jürgen Habermas (b. 1929) published his influential book *The Structural Transformation of the Public Sphere*. In his book he argued that what we now call "public opinion" originated in Britain during the late seventeenth century and that by the beginning of the eighteenth century we see the emergence of a public sphere "or reasoned discourses circulating in the political realm independently of both the Crown and Parliament" (McGuigan and Allan in Berry and Theobald, 2006: 92). Habermas defined the "public sphere" as

> a domain of our social life in which such a thing as public opinion can be formed ... Citizens act as a public when they deal with matters of general interest without being subject to coercion; thus with the guarantee that they may assemble and unite freely, and express and publicize their opinions freely. When the public is large, this kind of communication requires certain mean of dissemination and influence; today, newspapers and periodicals, radio and television are the media of the public sphere. (Habermas in Marris and Thornham, 1996: 92)

As Habermas put it, "it was private people who related to each other as a public" and that "new forms of public institution thus incorporated the private" (Habermas cit. in Baker: 321). There might be an argument here that the eventual rise of the fashion press represents one of these quintessential blendings of public and private. Printed for anyone who could purchase them, they also represent personal choices that were unlikely to remain private.

The coffee house provided the perfect medium, the pleasure of sipping such an exotic new beverage notwithstanding, for bringing together the well-to-do bourgeoisie for a friendly banter about the latest events, gossip, and fashion. But for an increasingly wider public, a more efficient means of communication was required and that was "the published word"; in other words, the "fourth estate," or the press.

The government was quick to curtail too much freedom for the press and acted accordingly. Thus, in 1712 a series of "taxes on knowledge" were implemented, the most important being the stamp tax (which was not completely eliminated until 1855) which enabled the Crown to control the right of publication and that attracted criticism, and on this occasion from high-profile writers. Habermas argued that "an extensive array of critical, if almost exclusively bourgeois voices were heard in the news journals. These voices were willing and able to take issue with the Crown's conduct and Parliament's legislative performance" (McQuigan and Allan in Berry and Theobald, 2006: 94).

If this challenging, often enraged temperament found its expression in publications such as John Tutchin's *Observer* (1702), Daniel Defoe's *The Review* (1704), and Jonathan Swift's *Examiner* (1710), for Habermas, it was Nicholas Amhurst's *Craftsman* (1726), together with Edward Cave's *Gentleman's Magazine* (1731), which signaled that "the press was for the first time established as a genuinely critical organ of a public engaged in critical political debate: as the fourth estate." Indeed, with the decline of the clubs and the coffee houses, the latter being a principal forum for the circulation of news (their golden age being between 1680 and 1730), the public was now largely being "held together" through an independent, market-based newspaper press subject to "professional criticism" (McQuigan and Allan in Berry and Theobald, 2006).

A publication fit for the educated few: The magazine

The English word "magazine" is derived from an Arabic term *makazin*, a storehouse, and by the 1600s had been adopted by the English to describe a warehouse for military shells and ammunition. Its first recorded use in a publishing context was in London in 1731, when it appeared in the title of the *Gentleman's Magazine*, promoted as a "store of useful information" (Parry, 2011: 165). Although the earliest magazines were published during the seventeenth century, it was during the Enlightenment that we see an impressive proliferation of periodicals, one of the reasons being that by their very nature they were able to specialize and to cater for a readership interested in learned subjects, such as science, philosophy, or literature. Consequently, they were often started and edited by well-known scholarly or literary personalities, among them Daniel Defoe, Jonathan Swift, and Thomas Addison, the reason being the emergence of a professional elite who were writers.

This was an era of rising prosperity and literacy. The expansion of professional elites was accompanied by a growth in confidence in scientific and professional expertise that the new periodicals were able to exploit by enrolling these professional groups as both writers and subscribers (Figure 2.5). These publications, in contrast to the newspapers, would draw on traditional founts of authority, expert writers, and discursive analysis (Petegree, 2014: 269). The expansion of the press was rapid. London had nine morning newspapers and ten evening ones, as well as six weeklies and three Sunday papers. Paris on the other hand had one daily, the *Journal de Paris*, in the old regime, but it also had its *almanachs* and pamphlets, which had emerged in the seventeenth century as a "kind of literature intended for the common people" (Chisick, 1991). Many included narratives, although less frequently until the 1770s, images of fashion. This is partly because the tax on paper meant that it was expensive to include images quite apart from the cost of having a wood-block, etching, or engraving designed by an artist.

Case study: Joseph Addison and *The Tatler*

Poet, playwright, and journalist Joseph Addison (1672–1719) became associated with the London elite coffee house culture. After working as a guide for the English aristocrats who embarked on the Grand Tour, he produced in collaboration with Richard Steele two magazines—*The Tatler* (1709–12) and *The Spectator* (1711–12, 1714) —"which did much to establish modern periodical journalism." Another important aspect of *The Tatler* was the use of a generous amount of advertising that promoted the commonplace aspects of life:

> *The Tatler* also vigorously pursued and gave a great deal of space to advertising: as many as 14 or 18 advertisements an issue, up to 150 a month. These promoted wigs, wheelchairs, birdcages, lotteries, cosmetics and medicines. As well as bringing valuable revenue they held up a mirror to the changing taste of London society. Readers could look to these for tips on correct deportment as well as bargains. (Pettegree, 2014: 276)

The Spectator continued the dual policy of its predecessor by publishing intellectual essays and articles but equally holding up a mirror to reflect the goings-on in London:

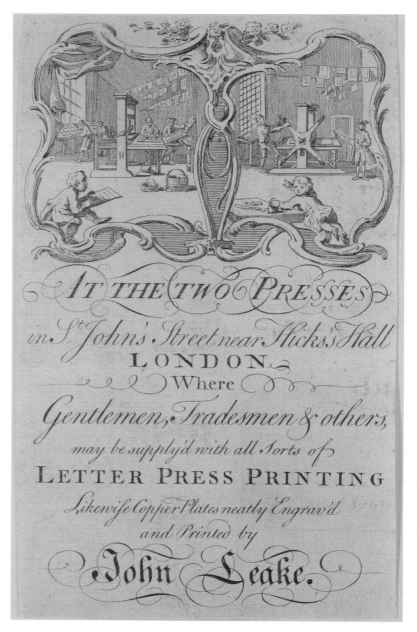

FIGURE 2.5 *"At the Two Presses in St. John's street near Hick's Hall, London where gentleman, tradesman, and others, may be supply'd with all sorts of letter press printing, likewise copper plates neatly engrav'd and printed by John Leake," c1760. Courtesy Lewis Walpole Library Yale University, trade tokens and bookplates, 1705–99 (bulk 1757–8), Quarto 66 726 T675.*

Advertised as the "sober reflections of a detached observer," Mr Spectator was never quite that; rather a wry, sometimes caustic and always penetrating observer of the foibles of London life. The enterprise was driven by the sheer brilliance of the writing, Addison and Steele ostensibly eschewed coverage of the news but the distinction was always more rhetorical than real. (Pettergree, 2014: 276–7)

Although the title of a series of articles entitled "Of the Pleasure of the Imagination" contributed by Addison and published in eleven installments in *The Spectator* in 1712 conjure up notions of esoteric philosophical debates, in fact this was not the case. Moreover, by focusing on taste— the central problem addressed in philosophical aesthetics, a new branch of philosophy which emerged during the Enlightenment—Addison became its premier arbiter in England, dealing with issues ranging from gardening and manners to literature and art. "The Pleasures of the Imagination" was his most influential piece of cultural journalism (Harrison, Wood and Gainger, 2000: 382). Its name has been evoked by a generation of cultural historians working from the 1980s onwards who examined anew the interrelationship of "middling-sort" (which preceded the concept of class) self-awareness, social life, and historical events (Brewer, 1997).

Taste was a subject sufficiently popular with the readership and belonged to an elite of the kind who spent their leisure time in coffee houses where they met like-minded clients and engaged in lively debates, the ideas spread further, driving many of the squibs and satires of the day (Figure 2.6). It was not only content that mattered, because Addison's style of writing was closer to journalism than academe.

These papers, written in his liveliest and most provocative manner, hardly formulated a systematic aesthetics, or pursued any problem very deeply, but they lived up to the author's claim to originality by posing most of the topics of eighteenth-century British aesthetics. In the paper announcing the series, Addison promises to "give some account" of "a fine taste in writing," which he defines as "that faculty of the soul which discerns the beauties of an author with pleasure, and the imperfections with dislike" (Beardsley, 1966: 185).

Two books on taste were published in 1757 by two British philosophers: David Hume's *Of the Standard of Taste* and Edmund Burke's *A Philosophical Enquiry into the Origin of our Ideas of the Sublime and the Beautiful,* in which they attempt to answer the question of whether we possess a special faculty which enables us to appreciate beautiful objects and reject ugly ones—and for both they answer in the affirmative. Hume argued that the blame in making a proper value judgment lies with the observer:

Some particular forms or qualities, from the original structure of the internal fabric are calculated to please, and others to displease; and if

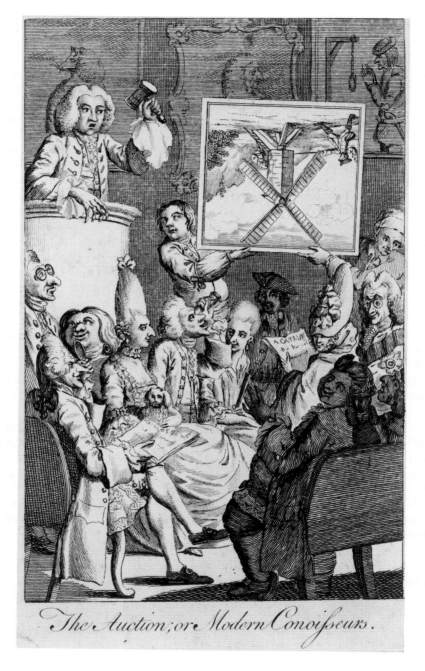

The Auction; or Modern Conoisseurs.

FIGURE 2.6 *"The Auction; or Modern Conoisseurs,"* The Oxford Magazine, *November 1771, engraving. Courtesy of the Library of Congress, Washington, D.C. Prints and Photographs Division Washington, D.C. PC 1—4770 (A size) [P&P].*

they fail of their effect in any particular instance it is from some apparent defect or imperfection of the organ. (Hume, 1965: 9)

Burke is more precise:

> But to cut off all pretence for cavilling, I mean by the word Taste no more than that faculty, or those faculties of the mind which are affected with, or which form a judgment of the works of imagination and the elegant arts ... And such principles of Taste, I fancy there are; however paradoxical it may seem to those, who on superficial view imagine, that there is so great a diversity of Tastes both in kind and degree, that nothing can be more indeterminate. (Burke, 1990: 13)

Taste was not only a philosophical subject of debate. The opposite was the case, because even more than subjects such as the "imagination" (itself a newcomer in philosophical debates, first introduced by Thomas Hobbes in *Leviathan* and defined as that special faculty needed in the creative process), "taste" became a faculty belonging to those who had an aesthetic experience, and not just for the artists.

Thus, if your "taste" was not good enough to appreciate Shakespeare or Reynolds, there was something wrong with you and not with the play or the painting, and the same held true regarding the choice of a new wallpaper, table, carriage, or the latest fashion in dress. It is at this point that "taste" becomes relevant to the world of fashion, a topic to which we will return in the section dedicated to the development of fashion magazines, or periodicals as they were at first called.

Images, as we have noted, were at first scarce among the printed word. They were costly and the tax on paper in England meant that their use was rationed. There were creative new forms of secular text and image in the mid- to late-eighteenth century that owed something to the religious tracts discussed previously. The importance of the printed trade card in generating esteem and reputation for a business in the eighteenth century is well established, although there are still questions as to how such cards were distributed, apart from those attached to objects such as furniture or mirrors or used for jotting memos and receipts (Scott, 2004; Berg and Clifford, 2007). Trade cards were a little bit like the flyers people used to put on cars to advertise a new club or a rave in the 1980s or the free cards available in many businesses today: many were beautifully illustrated by artists as famous as William Hogarth with the most up-to-date technology of printing, providing further information about new products in new places and how to use them (Figure 2.7). As well as sometimes being promotional, they also acted as *aides mémoires* about past purchases, and many were based on the familiar hanging shop-signs that began to be banned in England in the 1760s (Berg and Clifford, 2007: 151). Print and signatures could also convey the elegant aspiration of either a lady

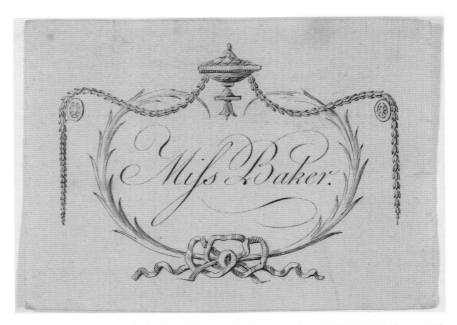

FIGURE 2.7 *"Miss Baker," calling card. Courtesy Lewis Walpole Library Yale University—boxed calling cards, LWL_4937_2.*

or a gentleman, illustrated here in the example of a neo-classical lady's "calling card" (Figure 2.8). The well-known flourish of a signature that accompanied much later twentieth-century column writing was in evidence as illustrative of a personality.

Women and writing

Many scholars have contended that the rise of the world of print as well as the growing spread of at least some fashion into the reach of most peoples in western Europe created new roles and spaces for women to write and to be published. Even the much-loved novelist Jane Austen has been reinterpreted as a brilliant critic of her day. In a book entitled *Jane Austen the Reader*, Olivia Murphy argues that Austen's fame is based upon her own reading of other's novels—"and the critical way in which she read them. She was a critical reader—investigating and evaluating literature, and articulating in her own works her version of what the novel could be" (Summary of Jane Austen the Reader, online, http://www.palgrave.com/gb/book/9781137292407 accessed 23 February 2016). This is a more expanded sense of what reviewing or "criticism" might mean, but it hits the mark, opening with a delightful quotation from *Northanger Abbey*:

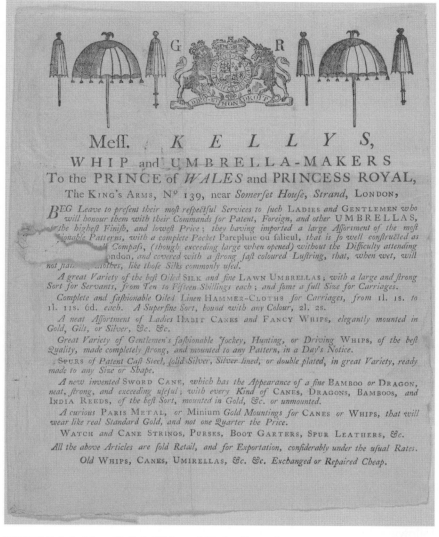

FIGURE 2.8 Mess. Kelly's Whip and Umbrella-Makers ... No. 139, near Somerset House, Strand, London [c 1795–1820], handbill, woodcut; 24 × 21 cm. Courtesy Lewis Walpole Library Yale University, 66 790 K29.

Let us leave it to the Reviewers to abuse such effusions of fancy at their leisure, and over every new novel to talk in threadbare strains of the trash with which the press now groans. (cit. in Murphy, 2013: 1)

Austen was alluding to the "Monthly and Critical Reviews" that were "until the nineteenth century, the two most important organs in Britain for the record and assessment of contemporary publications, both fiction and non-fiction" (Murphy, 2013: 2). Review journals attempted to note every new publication, and this, feminist scholars have noted, was in fact very good for women writers, whose work might otherwise have been ignored (Murphy, 2013: 2). Review writers by the nineteenth century tended to be turning to professionalism, rather than the amateur tradition of the previous century. Not everything could be reviewed anymore. Reviewers were paid in the well-known *Edinburgh Review* and *Quarterly Review*, which changed things once again (the academic reviewer today is generally *unpaid* for comments on other's academic projects such as books and journal articles, unless they are writing for a commercial art, design, or architecture magazine, which is hard for the public to understand). The nineteenth century was interested in the idea of women being reviewers, and women writers of the eighteenth century such as the *salonniers* Madame de Genlis and Madame de Staël had predicted the role—but male commentators were concerned that women might lack rules of judgment (Murphy, 2013: 25–6). It has been concluded that the nineteenth century was not a great time for the woman critic as the figure of the seventeenth-century "intellectual woman" was gradually obscured. Citing Simon Jarvis, Murphy notes that criticism should be considered in an expansive sense to embrace many genres in which women were active:

> Criticism, then, is not a genre, nor even a name for a group of genres. It happens not only in essays, reviews, philosophical dialogues, lecture courses, treatises; but also in novels, epigrams, plays and theatrical prologues and epilogues long poems, editions of texts, conversations, duels, gardens. (cit. in Murphy, 2013: 28–9)

Although Jarvis does not mention the fashion commentary or review, this might have been included in his embracing list, and his comments underline why in this work as well as *Fashion Writing and Criticism*, we referred to many formats *outside* the direct arena of sartorial fashions. Hence, our plea to students that they embrace as many formats as possible in developing their ideas, watching plays, looking at garden and interior design, and following debates.

Women, of course, continued to write, sometimes as professional journalists, including the American nineteenth-century celebrity journalist (Mary Katherine) Kate Field (1838–1896), supporter of black rights and founder of one of the first American women's clubs, seen here looking wistful in a photograph by Reutlinger (Figure 2.9). The profession of editing fashion magazines was generally occupied by women (Oscar Wilde at *The Woman's World* is a notable exception), as this "sex" was felt to possess the right understanding, access, and viewpoint to write about women's fashion. In France, the men's magazines that were published there were often influenced by queer men such as the balletomane Rolf de Maré, who

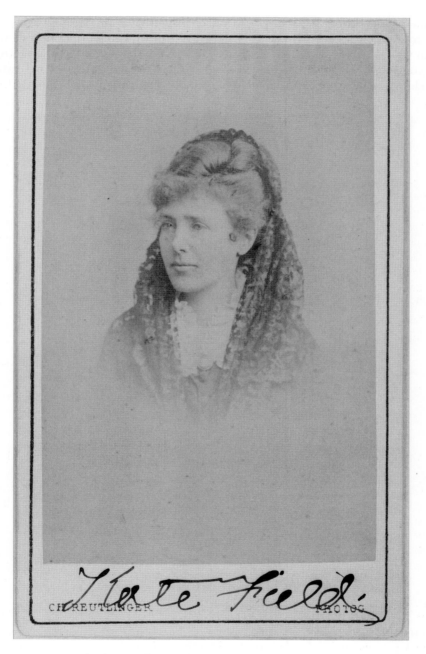

FIGURE 2.9 *Charles Reutlinger, photographer, "Kate Field [1838–1896]," Paris c1868, photographic print on carte de visite mount. Courtesy Library of Congress Prints and Photographs Division Washington, D.C. LOT 13301, no. 188 [P&P].*

funded the periodical *Monsieur*, managed by journalist and theatre producer Jacques Hébertot (Potvin, 2015: 242). Images of women journalists at work in the fashion field seem to be scarce, apart from the well-known scenes of women attending New Look and other postwar fashion parades. The "lady editors" tended to be formidable figures like Carmel Snow (Figure 2.10).

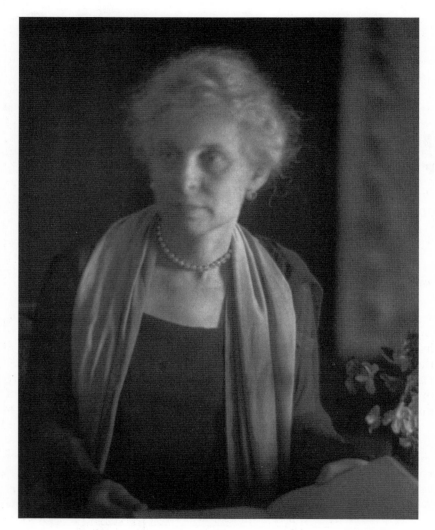

FIGURE 2.10 *Doris Ulmann, photographer, "Edna Woolman Chase, Editor Vogue,"* in A portrait gallery of American editors/being a group of XLIII likenesses by Doris Ulmann; with critical essays by the editors and an introduction by Louis Evan Shipman, *New York: W.E. Rudge, 1925, [plate] VI, [page 21], photogravure, 20.2 × 15.5 cm, on sheet 40.1 × 28 cm. Courtesy Library of Congress Prints and Photographs Division Washington, D.C. PN4871.U6 (Case Y) [P&P].*

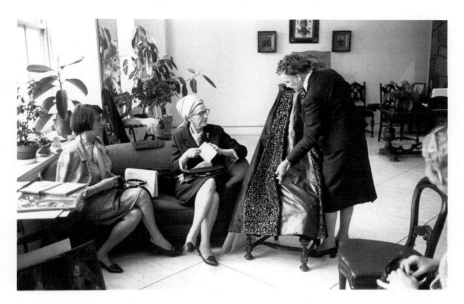

FIGURE 2.11 *Martha Swope, New York City Ballet—costumer Barbara Karinska shows costumes for "Don Quixote" to fashion writers, choreography by George Balanchine (New York) [probably 1965] Photo by Martha Swope. © New York Public Library for the Performing Arts, Billy Rose Collection.*
Karinska was a famous Russian-born costume designer for ballet and film, whereas a [costumer] today performs a technical role.

Wealthy editor and society figure Diana Vreeland complained that young women with a heavy tread should not be hired. She inspired and terrified in equal terms, helping to create much of the twentieth-century *mythos* of the field. Fleur Cowles, editor (also author and painter) of the short-lived *Flair* magazine (12 issues, February 1950–January 1951), lived grandly in an Albany, Picadilly (London) "set" (very exclusive apartment near the Burlington Arcade) and was the envoy from President Eisenhower to the Queen's Coronation. Images such as an (unnamed) late-middle aged journalist and her (unnamed) young female assistant at work interviewing costume designer Barbara Karinska in the 1960s about George Balanchine's production of *Don Quixote* (1965) indicate the strong gendered and class-inflected nature of much of the work (Figure 2.11). Women editors continue today to be unseated by men, as it is figures such as Anna Wintour of American *Vogue* who continue to dominate women's fashion magazines, although interestingly a probable majority of men are ascendant as stylists, special correspondents, and photographer-image makers in such magazines. In mid 2017 as we were completing this book, Alexandra Schulman, editor of British Vogue for twenty-five years, was unceremoniously removed and replaced by a man! He was also a man of colour, Edward Enninful, and the event was much reported upon.

3

A New Profession: The Journalist

The earliest journalists were a combination of printers, publishers, and occasional journalists all rolled into one. During the eighteenth century in England they both congregated and lived in Grub Street (today Milton Street, just north of Moorgate), which anticipated the famous Fleet Street, thus inaugurating the emergence of the "professional" (one writing for money) journalist. Grub street became associated with the idea of "hacks," who would do anything for money. The *Grub Street Journal* (established 1730) was a popular weekly devoted to satirical attacks on the new profession of journalism (Perry, 2011: 153).

By the mid-eighteenth century, many writers tried to make a living from books, magazines, and newspapers. One of its more famous examples was Samuel Johnson, later of *Oxford English Dictionary* fame. During the eighteenth century no fewer than twenty papers were published, but their circulation rarely exceeded 5,000 copies. Improvement of roads and the expansion of the General Post Office assisted the growth of the existing newspapers, and the ones printed in London achieved national status. Nevertheless, they were still too expensive, nor was there an adequate system of distribution; instead, coffee houses were used also as reading rooms: "at some points in the century, it was estimated that a single copy of a London newspaper could have as many as twenty individual readers" (Price, 1998: 422). It was the development of new technology as well as new audiences that facilitated the growth of this media, and consequently at the beginning of the nineteenth century we witness a rapid increase in publication of newspapers:

There had been daily newspapers, together with some evening papers, in London, and a number of weeklies which had appeared in the provinces. From 1780 onwards, evening papers appeared each day and Sunday newspapers were also produced. (Price, 1998: 423)

The broadsheet

The first nationally significant broadsheet—*The Times*—was published in 1785 as *The Daily Universal Register* and from January 1, 1788, as *The Times*, but it took several decades, until 1821, to see *The Sunday Times* first published.

In the second half of the nineteenth century, there was a great expansion of the periodical press, readers, and also infrastructure. Rosy Aindow has written an account of the great many "penny weeklies" and popular, cheap periodicals that reported on fashion and also published patterns—*Myra's* from London being one of the most famous demotic periodicals (Aindow: 44). *Myra's* dispensed with the eighteenth-century model of the fashion plate and peppered illustrations throughout its text (Breward cit. in Aindow: 44). Aindow cites the research of Cynthia White, who points out that new types of very cheap paper were produced in the 1880s via a Swedish wood-pulp innovation, and linotype (from 1889), making mechanical printing very cheap (Aindow: 45).

New distribution networks developed, some unsavory. In many countries, newspapers were distributed by under-age children on the streets and for negligible wages. A special photographic investigation in the United States by Lewis Hine commissioned by the anti-child labor organization the National Child Labor Committee (conducted between 1908 and 1924) yielded tragic images such as this (Figure 3.1), which makes one wonder what the "democratization" of print really meant—others suffered in the process.

New types of reading materials were also produced for use on train and subway journeys that had to be light, not too long and close to disposable. They were sold from kiosks on the platform and at exits on the street (Figure 3.2), sometimes even laid out on the street itself (Figure 3.3). This was a common sight in every busy commercial and residential street and railway station around the world until the contraction of this type of commerce in the past ten to twenty years (the "newsagent" today is likely to be making more profit from online and other gambling wins in Britain and Australia—some also sell stamps now that the state has closed many General Post Offices—another transaction that has declined dramatically with the use of email and social media to communicate).

The tabloids

While the history of each of the different means of communications had its own distinctive features, there was a year of convergence, notably 1896, which stands out in retrospect as a landmark date in the history of communications as a whole. It was a landmark because it anticipated the future, although it was not recognized as such at the time. This was the year

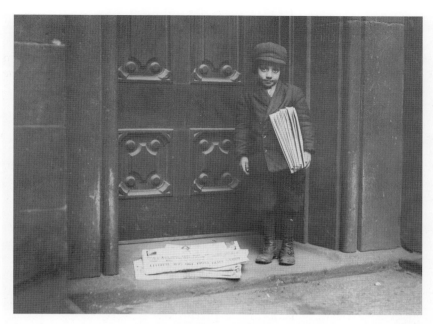

FIGURE 3.1 *Lewis Wickes Hine [attributed], Untitled ["newsboy"], [1913?], from album of street trades, possibly taken in either Pittsburgh or New York, glass negative, 5 × 7 in. Courtesy of the Library of Congress Prints and Photographs Division Washington, D.C. LOT 7480, v. 3, no. 3507-A [P&P] LC-H5- 3507-A.*

not only of the first London to Brighton car rally but of the founding of the *Daily Mail* and of the beginning of regular cinema shows in London's West End. This was also the year when the young Guglielmo Marconi arrived in London to display his bundle of wireless patents that he kept in a black box (Briggs, 1994: 243).

In 1896—borrowing the concept of popular journalism from the American Press—Alfred Harmsworth launched the first British tabloid, the halfpenny *Daily Mail*. Harmsworth, later Lord Northclife, himself an early motorist and future editor of a volume on *Motors and Motor Driving* (1902), promised the new readers of the *Daily Mail*, a popular newspaper to which the label of the "new journalism" was attached. Thus, the "four leading articles, a page of Parliament, and columns of speeches would NOT be found" in it. Lord Salisbury, England's Conservative Prime Minister at the end of the century, might have dismissed the *Daily Mail* as "a journal produced by office boys for office boys," but by then nearly a million copies of it were selling, and within the next decade Harmsworth was to take control of *The Times*, England's supreme "quality newspaper", as well (Briggs, 1994).

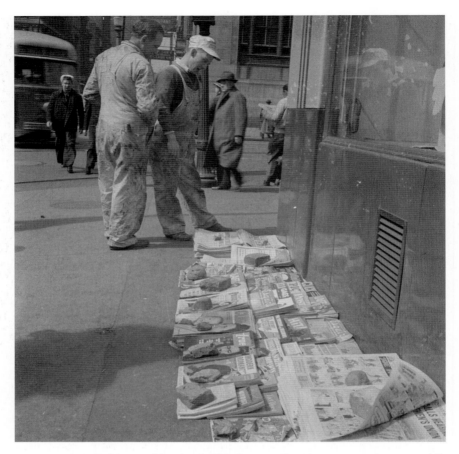

FIGURE 3.2 *Baltimore, Maryland, "Workers reading the newsstand papers while waiting for a trolley after work." Courtesy of the Library of Congress Prints and Photographs Division Washington, DC, LC-DIG-fsa-8d27929 (digital file from original neg.) LC-USW3-022102-E (b&w film nitrate neg.)*

Not only was this new format (tabloid) newspaper cheaper (it cost half a penny while broadsheets cost at least a penny), but their most radical characteristic was the new approach to storytelling, which typically included the leader-page articles, magazine items, half a column of society gossip, and a serialized story. This was the busy man's newspaper, not taking too long to read, and even more importantly, women found in it quite a few issues of interest. A satirical cartoon from the late nineteenth century concerning the newspaper *The Age* ("price 4 d.") depicts the bard Shakespeare in the middle reading drama and theatricals, surrounded by a range of figures reading their own particular interests; a fop reads "court and fashion general intelligence," a group of middle-class women read the "best family

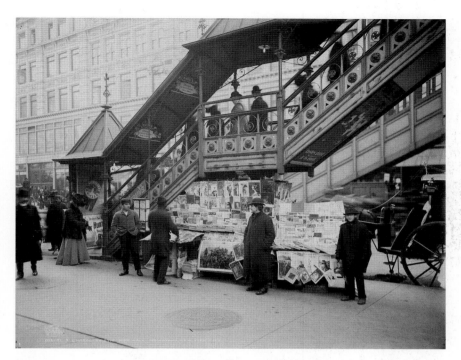

FIGURE 3.3 *A characteristic sidewalk newstand [*sic], *New York City, late December 1902–January 1903, Detroit Publishing Co., glass negative; 8 × 10 in. Gift; State Historical Society of Colorado; 1949. Courtesy of the Library of Congress Prints and Photographs Division Washington, DC LC-D4-16161 [P&P].*

The New York City location seems to be 23rd Street just east of Sixth Avenue, Manhattan. Stairs probably lead to "El" elevated transit line. Visible magazines on display are from late December 1902 and January 1903.

journal ... novels and tales," and various male types read either sporting news, literature, cotton reports, or science and philosophy (Figure 3.4). News was diversifying and addressing different audiences; the cartoon does not necessarily suggest one is superior to the other, although Shakespeare is the only human figure represented who does not look ridiculous, and he looks rather world-weary.

Encouraged by its success, Lord Northcliffe launched in 1903 a second tabloid: the *Daily Mirror*, on this occasion aimed mostly at a women's readership. Its aims and objectives were described as "a newspaper for gentlewomen by gentlewomen," and although it was proclaimed to be a success, it failed. One simple reason was that as a daily newspaper the *Daily Mirror* tried to adopt the format of weekly and monthly fashion and consumer journalism and women needed only so much information about the latest Paris fashions. Another even more serious criticism was that its readers, mostly middle-class women, could not identify with the lifestyle

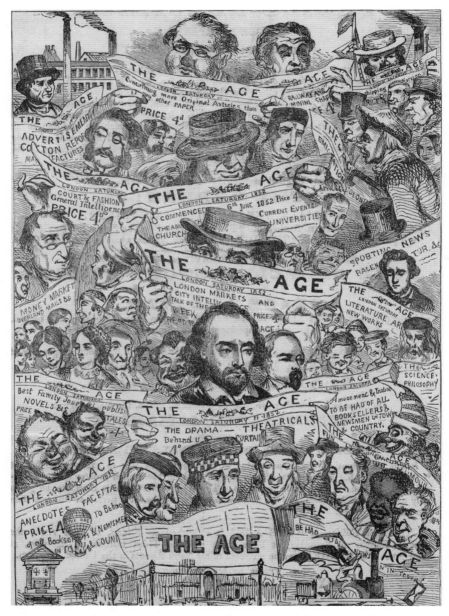

FIGURE 3.4 *Ebenezer Landells (1808–1860), printmaker.* "The Age," *circa June 1852 (date taken from a page in the illustration), print on wove paper: wood engraving; sheet 18.9 × 12.9 cm. Courtesy Lewis Walpole Library, Yale University, 852.06.01.01.*

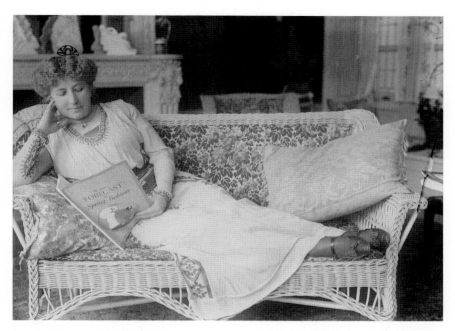

FIGURE 3.5 *"Mme. Gadski," Bain News Service [1916], glass negative: 5 × 7 in. Courtesy of the Library of Congress Prints and Photographs Division Washington, D.C. LC-B2- 3774-4-x [P&P].*

Photograph shows opera singer Johanna Gadski (1872–1932) reading copy of Vogue *magazine ("Forecast of Spring Fashions") dated February 1, 1916.*

content based on reporting from Parisian fashion houses which catered for an altogether different lifestyle meant for the wealthy grand bourgeoisie. Madame Gadsky, an Opera singer, here depicted reading the *Vogue* forecast of Spring fashions, was clearly a New York lady who at home, at least, was a lady of leisure (Figure 3.5). She would not have been photographed reading the *Mirror*.

In 1904, just before its closure, the *Daily Mirror* sacked its women's editorial team and was re-launched as the *Daily Illustrated Mirror*. It is this type of news organ for everyday people that is satirized in the 1914 North American print "Fashion Notes," in which a group of ruddy-cheeked and shabbily dressed working-class women gather on some park benches marked "reserved for ladies" and listen aloud as fashion news is read out (Figure 3.6). As they carry parcels the suggestion is that they are hardly 'ladies' ('ladies' in this period preferred to have parcels delivered; the parcels also might carry suggestions of piecework—parts of clothes, etc. to be sewn at home—or fine washing) and the class- based snobbery is well made. Such a satire is also likely a critique of the global suffrage movement, with the

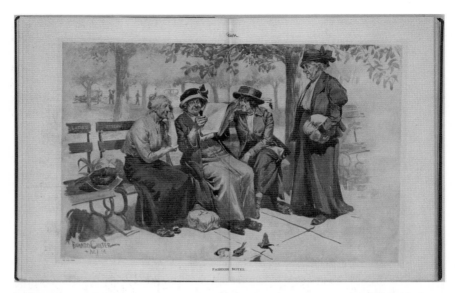

FIGURE 3.6 *Richard Culter,* Fashion notes, Puck, *vol. 75, no. 1933 (March 21, 1914), centerfold. New York: Published by Puck Publishing Corporation, 295–309 Lafayette Street, March 21, 1914, photomechanical print: offset. Courtesy of the Library of Congress Prints and Photographs Division Washington, D.C., AP101.P7 1914 (Case X) [P&P].*

suggestion that the sensibly dressed and rather mannish women have no ear for any real news but fashion news. It also might be a joke about the (uneven) spread or success of mass-produced fashions in the society that was creating the best-dressed nation of women in the world, the United States. The feminist Rozika Bédy-Schwimmer (better known as Rózsa Schwimmer) (1877–1948) collected an image of women reading newspapers together (possibly in Hungary in 1913, the year before she visited the United States on a lecture tour), the significance of which is hard to assess, but it indicates the importance of the press in creating voices and platforms for women in public space (Figure 3.7).

Fashion journalism therefore required a different approach from the general news, and how this was pursued with success will be analyzed in Part II of this book.

The academic world and the media

By way of concluding this section, we need to consider where, when, and why did media become a university subject, such that you might be studying it now? This took place firmly during the 1960s, at the same time

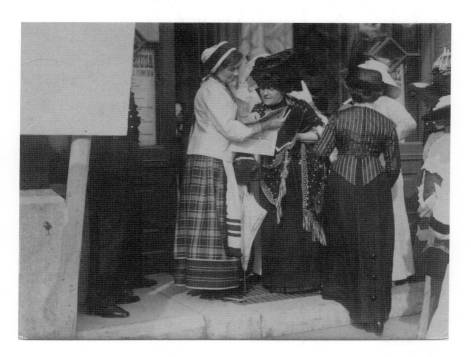

FIGURE 3.7 *Women reading a newspaper on a street corner, 1913, Rosika Schwimmer Papers. The New York Public Library, Manuscripts and Archives Division.*

Schwimmer was a Hungarian pacifist-feminist who worked as a correspondent for several European newspapers and was nominated for the Nobel Peace Prize in 1946. She toured the USA in 1914–15 and later tried to settle there, but was accused of being a socialist.

as a spate of new subjects—among them the controversial subject of media studies—emerged in the United Kingdom at the end of the 1950s—allegedly inaugurating inter-disciplinarity as their chosen methodology, resulting in two distinct strands in the British Academic world. The first pertained to "social science (sociology, social psychology, political communications)," the second to "the humanities (notably English literary study)" (Marris and Thornham, 1999: 5). They reflect in the first instance the ideological position of the "Frankfurt School", while the second strand was responding to a native source of influence, "Leavisism"—connected to the Faculty of English and the so-called Leavisites at the University of Cambridge (Marris and Thornham, 1999: 8). The Leavisites took a particular approach to the study of literary texts that privileged overarching themes and grand human narratives: theirs was an approach firmly rejected by post-structuralism and post-modernism of the 1980s and 1990s, which argued that the Leavises had privileged canonical texts and great white men.

But the new academic discipline of media studies did not invent inter-disciplinarity as a new methodology. That accolade goes to a group of left-wing German intellectuals who came to be known as the "Frankfurt School," which started its existence in 1923 as the "Frankfurt Institute of Social Research" and became known as the "Frankfurt School of Critical Theory." In 1930, a professor of philosophy was appointed to its directorship: Max Horkheimer. In his inaugural speech given one year later, he outlined the importance of introducing an interdisciplinary approach to critical theory, whereby scientific research would be combined with Marxist social theory by producing a synthesis between Sigmund Freud's latest research in psychoanalysis and Marxism. Horkheimer collaborated on this new program with fellow philosophers Herbert Marcuse, Erich Fromm, and Theodor Adorno. With the election of Adolf Hitler as Chancellor of Germany in 1933 the "Frankfurt School" was forced to relocate first to Geneva, and one year later, at the invitation of Columbia University, the Institute traveled to the United States, where they were able to continue to function until the end of World War II, when some of its members returned to Germany. The "Frankfurt School" reopened in 1950 with the addition of important new members such as Jürgen Habermas, where it still functions to this day (Payne in Payne, 1997: 205).

At about the same time in England, we see the emergence of a radical new approach to teaching English literature at universities, which had its roots at the beginning of the nineteenth century when the study of English was a Church of England monopoly. As such, Oxford and Cambridge Universities—which introduced it as an academic subject—were forced to comply with their requirements of focusing on the study of the English language. Fortunately, this monopoly was broken by the founding of a London college: King's College (later London University College), where focus was shifted from language to literary studies.

A chair of English was established at Oxford in 1894, but it still had to contain an important element of historical language study, including Anglo-Saxon, Gothic, etc. Things were easier in Cambridge, where a School of English was established as recently as 1911, and by 1920s important reforms could be introduced in the curriculum. The engineers of this change were a group of people who began teaching at Cambridge in the 1920s: A. Richards, William Empson, and F. R. Leavis.

Richards pioneered a new method in criticism still in use today, known as "close reading," whereby his students focused exclusively on what is "on the page" and ignored the historical and cultural context which produced the literary work. Thus, instead of worrying about Charles Dickens's biographical details or the unequal Victorian society that prompted him to write novels about social injustice, what mattered was simply analysis of the text! Richards called his method **"Practical Criticism"**, which was also the title of his seminal book on the subject published in 1929. Not everybody agreed with his technique: "T.S. Eliot called it the lemon-squeezer school of criticism, and his own critical writing is always on a much more generalized level" (Barry, 2001: 15).

It was Frank Raymond Leavis and his wife Queenie Dorothy Leavis who are particularly relevant to media and journalism studies because of their pioneering interests in journalism and popular fiction respectively. The former wrote his doctoral thesis on literature and journalism while Queenie was interested in popular fiction. In 1932, they founded together the influential magazine *Scrutiny*. In his book *Mass Civilization and Minority Culture* (1930) published by the Minority Press (a small publishing house founded by one of Leavis's former students, Gordon Fraser), F. R. Leavis wrote that British culture was undergoing a crisis because it was under the threat of being "Americanized" and similarly Queenie was equally disapproving of what she called "pulp fiction," which reflected the general process of "dumbing down" (a term which originated in 1933 in the movie business needing to cater for a majority who did not have high levels of education).

F. R. and D. Q. Leavis were not alone in their disdain of popular culture and mass media; they concurred with the position taken by the members of the "Frankfurt School" targeted especially at *art engagé* (engaged art), such as Bertolt Brecht's political plays.

In their seminal book *The Dialectic of Enlightenment* first published in 1944, Max Horhkeimer and Theodor Adorno devoted a chapter entitled "The Culture Industry: Enlightenment as Mass Deception" to popular forms of entertainment such as the cinema, radio, and magazines, which they argued had become an industry motivated by financial gain, which threaten "authentic culture."

Frank and Queenie Leavis too argued that "the culture industry" (Hollywood, the mass media, the record industry) was increasingly organized like any other commercial sector of manufacture and consumption, and culture had become commodified. In contrast to the authenticity of folk and popular art and the human insights of genuine high art, the culture industry supplied "substitute gratification," and promoted the cult of personality and other authoritarian attitudes. Leisure was rationalized like industrial production, and consciousness was integrated smoothly into the cycle of capitalist reproduction and accumulation (Lazarfield and Merton in Marris and Thornham, 1999: 7). The battle between high and low culture was taking a new form and it was central to academic debate.

F. R. Leavis's new approach to literary theory was adopted in the 1960s by a group of academics influenced by Leavis's ideas, among them Raymond Williams, Stuart Hall, and Richard Hoggart, founders of British Cultural Studies, distinct from the ideology which informed the more general "Cultural Studies" because of its Marxist approach. In 1964, Stuart Hall founded the most influential *The New Left Review* and during the same year he became a member of the CCCS (Centre of Contemporary Cultural Studies) affiliated to Birmingham University.

Toward the end of the twentieth century the rapid development of technology, globalization, the "Fall of the Berlin Wall" in 1989, and the end of the "Cold War" contributed to a radical new way of approaching media studies at university level. As observed by Marris and Thornham, the "mass" in the term "mass media" was eliminated; instead, we have the "new media" center stage for the new millennium.

Thus, the term "media" in "media studies" brings with it the ideas of channels of communication, complex technologies of mechanical or electronic reproduction, and means of expression. Since the 1980s there have been accelerating developments in microelectronics, computing, telecommunications, and digital software, which have made for new kinds of electronic technologies of reproduction and dissemination, new channels of communication, and new means of expression. These are appropriately often referred to as "new media," and studying their social and cultural role is properly the province of media studies fitted to comprehend and explain contemporary practices (1999: 782). The analysis of the relationship of old and new media is one of the aims of this book.

PART TWO

Understanding Fashion Journalism

4

Fashion Journalism: History

In the "late" July 1916 issue of American *Vogue*, its editor Max Eastman posed the rhetorical question: "What is the matter with magazine writing?," and in the time-honored tradition of oratory—he proceeded to answer the question himself:

> What will you pay me per word? said I. And in that question I stated better than 2,000 words can tell, what is the matter with magazine writing. Magazine writing is professional. It is work and not play. And for that reason it is never profoundly serious or intensely frivolous enough to captivate the soul. It lacks abandon. It is simply well done. Amazingly well done. To me the quantity and fluency and consummate skill of American magazine writing is a perpetual miracle. (Max Eastman: "What is the Matter with Magazine Writing (An attempt at a sympathetic diagnosis)," *Vogue* (American) Late July Issue, 1916, p. 77)

Eastman went on to note:

> In order to please everybody and offend none, he must eliminate all these warm and spontaneous impulses that are his very own, whatever they be, and confine his efforts to the creation of superficially and obviously pleasant qualities, like fluency and wit, and the glamour of sexuality and money and a few touches of pathos and purity and no difficulties for the understanding. (Eastman, 1916, p. 83)

One hundred years later, Max Eastman's words ring so true that his advice to the magazine journalist would be as valid of the twenty-first-century journalist as it was when he offered it.

How did it all begin?

A new subject of interest: Manners and mores

The French fashion press appeared just after the first half of the eighteenth century. But clothes did not appear for the first time in print in this century, far from it, as pointed out by fashion historian Lou Taylor, who placed the earliest publications of specialized books on dress during the High Renaissance:

> Between 1520 and 1610 over 200 collections of engraving, etchings and woodcuts were published in Germany, Italy, France and Holland, concerning clothes and personal adornment. (Taylor, 2004: 5)

Nor was publication of these books the result of a special interest in sartorial fashion or the latest "look" worn in Paris, Venice, or elsewhere; rather, the reason was anthropological, to do with the manners, mores, and newly discovered faraway cultures.

Details of the "strange" manners, "habits," and clothing of distant peoples were published with minimal descriptive texts and with plates redrawn from travelers', traders', and missionary tales. The wealthy consumers of such books, their heads filled with vague visions of the "Hindoo" and a fantastical mysterious land called "Cathay," often had little notion of where these exotic people lived. "So vague were contemporary notions of what constituted the geography and history of the 'East Indies', noted John Irwin, that many were unaware of India and China having separate civilisations" (Taylor, 2004). Daniel Roche even provides a statistic of all the books on clothes published in France between the sixteenth and the eighteenth centuries: thus, before 1600, eight books on clothes were published, and between 1750 and 1799, ninety-eight books were published; but to this dry piece of information he adds a charming comment regarding their increasing popularity:

> Costume and its diverse representations thus took place in the gallery of marvels of nature and prodigies of human creation. (Roche, 1994: 12)

The starting point: François Desprez and Cesare Vecellio

One of the earliest examples analyzed by Roche is François Desprez's book published in 1562 with the impressive title *Recueil de la diversité des habits qui sont à présent en usage tant en pays d'Europe, Asie, Afrique* ("Collection of the diversity of clothes at present in use in the countries of Europe as well as Asia and Africa"). The book included 120 engravings accompanied by *quatrains*. Desprez chose his subjects from a variety of sources: people from all walks of life, from all countries, and we find among the plates "The Italian Woman," "The Citizen of Paris," "The Old Citizen," "The Knight of the Order of the Gentlemen." We find "foreigners"—"the Englishwoman," "the Woman of Picardy"—and stranger still we find *des bizzareries*—"The Standing Monkey" or "The Cyclops."

The accompanying *quatrains* are mostly explanatory but often humorous stereotyping of the customs and costumes from other countries as described in travelers' tales: here comes the Englishwoman:

> See how her square cap is lined with furs
> She is still easy to recognize
> though we can hardly see
> into it, so great is its size. (Roche, 1994: 12)

In 1590, the first edition of a splendid book was published in Venice: Cesare Vecellio's *Degli Habiti Antichi et Moderni di Diverse Parti Del Mondo* (*The Clothing, Ancient and Modern, of Various Parts of the World*) followed in 1598 by a second expanded edition. The book became a resounding success because it had no precedent regarding its breadth, given that it covered not only clothing in Italy across a time span from the Antiquity to contemporary fashions but also from other European countries and continents, including Africa and Asia, and for the 1598 edition, the Americas:

> As a writer, too, Vecellio calls attention to the breadth and variety of the styles of dress he shows in his woodcuts. In his titles and his preface he emphasizes the immense efforts he has put into gathering clothing from "the various nations of the world" including places so far away that it has been difficult to acquire trustworthy information about them … Vecellio offers more information about nearby and faraway costume and custom than any of the dozen costume books published before him. (Rosenthal and Jones, 2006: 8)

So how did Vecellio, who never left his native Veneto—with the exception of a short visit to Germany—get his information? To start with—like his famous cousin the painter Titian (Tiziano Vecellio)—he would have been familiar with the work of Venetian painters both past and present, especially Quattrocento narrative painters like Gentile Bellini, Vittore Carpaccio, and Giovanni Mansueti, who provided a visual source for the study, not only of costume in Venice, but also its streets and people. They were among the first to depict also the exotic costume of its multicultural inhabitants and visitors. But what makes Vecellio's book special is that alongside visual images he provided detailed explanatory texts not only regarding the outfit represented on the page but also about its wearers, their identity, social class, and what it all meant; in other words, an early "Wikipedia." Vecellio would also have been familiar not only with François Desprez's *Recueil* but with other books such as Ferdinand Bertellis's *Omnium fere Gentium Nostrae Aettatis Habitus* (*The Clothing of almost All the Peoples of Our Age*) published in Venice in 1563 (Rosenthal and Jones, 2006: 43, note 24, see also Paulicelli, 2014 in: *Writing Fashion in Early Modern Italy: From Sprezzatura to Satire*, particularly on Castiglione and Vecellio.

It was during the seventeenth century that we witness the emergence of visual representations of contemporary ways of dressing, and as James Laver observed in the postwar period, we can find them in the engravings of Abraham Bosse and the etchings of Jacques Callot (Laver, 1969: 104).

Vecellio's model of depicting the dress of foreign climes with class (or status as it tended to be at that time), region, and occupation was extremely influential, and continued to be used well into the nineteenth century: an elegant eighteenth-century example was compiled by the Jesuit J. B. du Halde illustrating China, Tibet, and Korea and published in French in 1735 (Figures 4.1 and 4.2). Such images fell under the incipient category of what we might now call "human geography."

The antecedents of the fashion magazine

In 1665, an unusual magazine was published in France—the *Journal des Sçavans*—and what was unusual about it was the breadth of scholarly subjects included. This was a major innovation in the European book trade: a journal devoted primarily to discoveries in the arts and sciences, with some additional notifications, for legal customers, of decisions taken by the civil and ecclesiastical courts. It was set to appear weekly, on the grounds that novelties lost their lustre if held back for a monthly or annual publication. "The volume was also provided with a full scholarly apparatus: tables, notes, index, and cumulative bibliography" (Pettegree, 2014: 270).

The magazine became also the template for subsequent scholarly journals and its influence was immediately felt across the channel with publication of the *Philosophical Transactions*, whose editors were members of the newly founded Royal Society.

> The *Philosophical Transactions* was nevertheless a more elitist venture than the *Journal des Sçavans*. The 300 copies printed of the *Transactions* were more than enough for the fellows, and the Society made little attempt to spread its reach beyond the circle of experts. Both periodicals, however, were self-consciously behind a part of the international community of learning and discovery: the Republic of Letters celebrated in Pierre Bayle's monumental and long-running review journal *Nouvelles de la République Des Letters (1684–1718)*. The first issue of the *Philosophical Transactions* contained one article contributed from France, and another from Italy; subsequent numbers frequently carried articles translated from the *Journal des Sçavans* (Pettegree, 2014: 272).

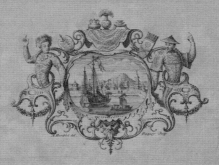

DESCRIPTION
GEOGRAPHIQUE
HISTORIQUE, CHRONOLOGIQUE,
POLITIQUE, ET PHYSIQUE
DE L'EMPIRE DE LA CHINE
ET
DE LA TARTARIE CHINOISE,

ENRICHIE DES CARTES GENERALES ET PARTICULIERES
de ces Pays, de la Carte générale & des Cartes particulieres du Thibet, & de
la Corée, & ornée d'un grand nombre de Figures & de Vignettes gravées
en Taille-douce.

Par le P. J.B. DU HALDE, *de la Compagnie de* JESUS.

TOME SECOND.

A PARIS,
Chez P. G. LE MERCIER, Imprimeur-Libraire, rue Saint Jacques,
au Livre d'Or.

M· DCC· XXXV.
AVEC APPROBATION ET PRIVILEGE DU ROY.

FIGURE 4.1 *J. B. Du Halde,* Description Geographique, Historique, Chronologique, Politique, et Physical de l'Empire de la Chine et de la Tartarie Chinoise, *vol. 2, Paris: Le Mercier, 1735, frontispiece. Courtesy Lewis Walpole Library, Yale University.*

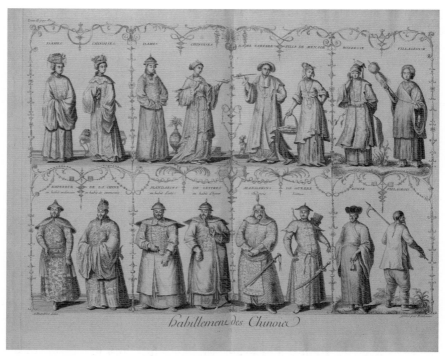

FIGURE 4.2 *"Habillemens des Chinois" (folding plate), in J. B. Du Halde,*
Description Geographique, Historique, Chronologique, Politique, et Physical de
l'Empire de la Chine et de la Tartarie Chinoise, *vol. 2, Paris: Le Mercier, 1735.*
Courtesy Lewis Walpole Library, Yale University.

The *Mercure Galant,* founded by the writer Jean Donneau de Visé, was
published in France from 1672, but because of the connotations of frivolity
associated with the title, few realized that it superseded the "high-minded
Journal des Sçavans" (Pettegree, 2014: 274). Moreover, unlike the latter, the
Mercure Galant had its origins in a different tradition, that of the "gallant"
satirical and literary press. Instead of focusing on the latest developments in
the sciences and the arts, the *Mercure Galant* covered subjects of popular
interest, among them fashion, and although it was not the first fashion
magazine (this will be published a century later), the *Mercure Galant* was the
first magazine to pay attention to it. Gallant journalism often used the device
of the letter; it allowed a well-bred tone that promoted a feeling of sympathy
between reader and writer. The latter made confidences and observations,
repeated the gossip of the salons, and used various means to make his fictions
sound like fact so as to win his readers' confidence, give an air of authenticity
to his information, and provoke imitation (Roche, 1994: 479).

   "Gallant journalism" created its own journalists fit for purpose: the
gallant journalists who "only referred to fashion by reason of an external

and wholly social legitimation since it had not yet achieved recognition and totally autonomous expression" (Roche, 1994). De Visé, himself a writer, was already involved with such scholarly events as the famous *querrelle des anciens et des Modernes* (quarrel between the ancients and moderns). This disputation, which rocked the French Academy controlling learning, was the consequence of a meeting in 1687 when Charles Perrault (1628–1703)— founder of a new literary genre, the fairy tale (best loved by young and old alike for such enchanting stories as "Cinderella," "Little Red Riding Hood," and "Sleeping Beauty")—proclaimed the superiority of the moderns over the ancients. But what really sparked the debate was his comparison of the reign of Louis XIV with that of the Roman Emperor Augustus in Rome, whom Perrault considered not superior to the famous "Sun King":

> Beautiful Antiquity has always been an object of veneration
> but I do not believe that it has ever been worthy of adoration.
> I look upon the Ancients without bending the knee;
> they were great it is true, but they were men just like us;
> without fear of being unjust we may compare
> the century of Louis with the century of Augustus. (quoted in: Harrison, Wood and Gaiger, 2000: 15)

Central to the quarrel was the notion that art, like science, is based on rational principles established during Antiquity, and although a wealth of treatises on rhetoric and poetry survived, this was not the case with the visual arts. As a consequence, a number of seventeenth-century writers such as Franciscus Junius took it upon themselves to rectify the situation by publishing treatises about the practice of the visual arts in which they prioritized reason over creativity:

> At the heart of the *doctrine classique* lay the conviction that reason was the instrument both of artistic creativity and of rational reflection. The true imitation of nature demanded that the artist not merely copy the external features presented by the natural world, but also penetrate through to the essential. The production of a work of art is guided by a set of eternally valid rules whose original apprehension is owed to the Ancients, but whose enduring validity is authorized by reason itself. (Harrison, Wood, and Gaiger, 2000: 16)

The *Mercure Galant* played an important part in the quarrel by aligning itself with the moderns, supported by luminaries as the playwright Jean Racine against the ancients. But what made the magazine special was the fact that Donneau de Visé adopted a pioneering agenda by inserting into it popular subjects, one of which was fashion.

Thus, the magazine was not only able to give the readers an idea about the latest fashions by using fashion plates but pioneered an early form of advertising by giving the name and Paris address of the *marchande des modes* who could supply each of the individual items needed to create the outfit (Morini 2006: 29). De Visé had a great deal of difficulty creating these fashion advertisements as the guilds (groups who controlled production) would not cooperate with someone who also had a type of secondhand shop (Françoise Tétart-Vittu, "The Fashion Print: An Ambiguous Object," in Norberg and Rosenbaum, 9–10). Other *journalistes* tried to compile lists of fashion merchants addresses and also ran into similar problems: "Like a good journalist, he [Donneau] praised himself: 'Paris and foreign countries want to learn about new fashions. The new fashions generally appear at the change of season; with the four 'extraordinary' editions [of the *Mercure Galant*] we will have all the fashions of the current year" (Tétart-Vittu 10). The famous fashion prints of the time were exported as far as China and the Indies (Tétart-Vittu; 11) (Figure 4.3). In the March 1678 issue of its new version entitled *Le Nouveau Mercure Galant*—which followed the first volume that lasted only one year (1677–8)—we find an illustration reproducing the interior of a shop selling fashion accessories accompanied by explanations of the items on display for the benefit of the clients. This was an unusual image that was not repeated due to the difficulties with the guilds mentioned above. After the death of its founder in 1710 the magazine changed ownerships and titles several times until 1724 when it became the *Mercure de France* (Morini, 2006). The historian David Pullin has pointed out that there is a strange hiatus between the visual energy (albeit within the rather restricted template of a figure generally situated on a blank background or within an interior) of the late seventeenth-century French magazine and the sudden rise of illustrated fashion periodicals in the 1770s that has never been fully explained (Pullin, *Reviews in History*, accessed 2016).

The fashion doll—Bringer of news

The emergence of a specialized fashion press is dated 1750,

> which although mostly French, quickly spread beyond its boundaries and helped reshape the dress of the European elites who were its readers, in line with French worldly sensibilities, just as their conduct and culture had previously been influenced by the luminaries of French philosophy, whose ideas had circulated through the increasingly numerous channels provided by books and the press (Roche, 1994: 470).

A precedent of the specialized fashion magazine were the fashion dolls of various sizes, some quite large, that were sent across Europe and even to colonial North America, and the costume historian François Boucher attributed the international success of French attire in the eighteenth century to the women who made the fashion dolls:

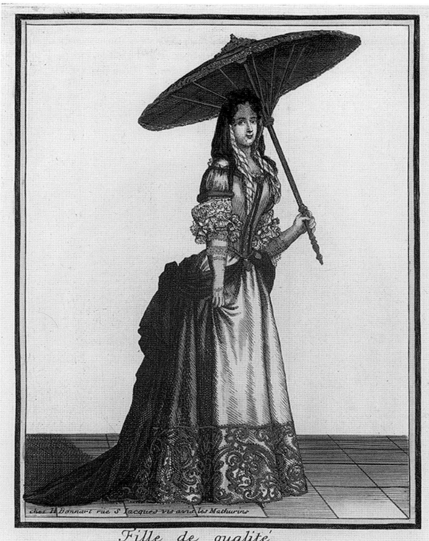

Fille de qualité

Ie mes a couuert mon visage   Par quelque rousseur n'endomage
De peur que l'ardeur du soleil   La beauté de mon teint vermeil .

FIGURE 4.3 *Henri Bonnart,* Fille de Qualité, *in "Recueil des modes de la cour de France," Hand-colored engraving on paper, Paris, 1680. Sheet: 14 3/8 × 9 3/8 in. (36.51 × 23.81 cm); composition: 10 3/4 × 7 3/4 in. (27.31 × 19.69 cm). Los Angeles County Museum of Art. Purchased with funds provided by The Eli and Edythe L. Broad Foundation, Mr. and Mrs. H. Tony Oppenheimer, Mr. and Mrs. Reed Oppenheimer, Hal Oppenheimer, Alice and Nahum Lainer, Mr. and Mrs. Gerald Oppenheimer, Ricki and Marvin Ring, Mr. and Mrs. David Sydorick, the Costume Council Fund, and members of the Costume Council (M.2002.57.21).*

The "universality" of French costume in the eighteenth century was largely the work of women. In France they controlled everything, King and country, the royal will and public opinion. But most of all, they were increasingly mistresses in their own homes. In all the capitals of Europe they waited impatiently for the arrival of the "doll from the rue Saint Honoré." (Boucher 1997: 318)

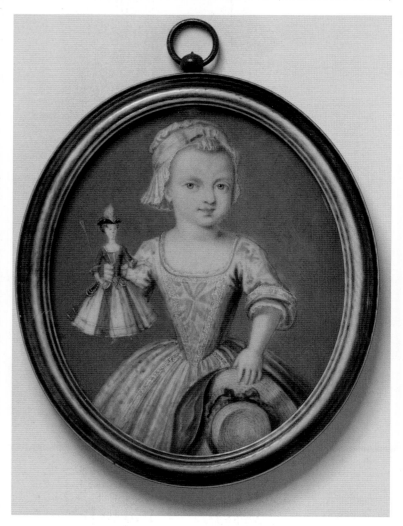

FIGURE 4.4 *Bernard Lens,* Portrait of Katherine Whitmore, *miniature, 1724, watercolor on ivory, Victoria and Albert Museum P.14-1971. © Victoria and Albert Museum, London.*

Katherine Whitmore's family came from Shropshire and her father was a Member of Parliament for Bridgnorth. The image shows her with the type of doll that likely also served as fashion information.

There is still debate surrounding surviving eighteenth-century dolls as to whether they are meant to be fashion advertisements, some form of entertainment, or for the use of children or adults (Figure 4.4). Probably, the use was a little of both, and a discarded fashion doll would make a good plaything.

The inter-war German researcher Max von Boehn gave a special role to the doll in terms of the dissemination of fashion: "At a time when as yet the press was non-existent, long before the invention of such mechanical means of reproduction as the woodcut and copperplate, to the doll was given the task of popularizing French fashions abroad" (Boehn, 1966: 136). Most of the surviving dolls are relatively small.

Neither word of mouth nor the lovable fashion dolls alone were fully effective in conveying fashion news, and when the fashion magazines emerged, they enjoyed instant success:

> From the beginning the publication of fashion journals could be presented as an almost guaranteed success, compared to these expensive, delicate and in the last analysis not very convenient artificial figures periodically presented to an admiring world. (Roche, 1994: 475)

The costume and fashion plate

Daniel Roche makes a distinction between plates representing "costume" and those representing "fashion," starting with representations of the latter either as collections of engravings or individual fashion plates. In them "text and illustration were effectively combined to make the changes, if not the newest styles, widely known." Subsequently two distinct categories of plates emerged: those of costume, aiming to "portray the diversity of past customs or national dress," while the latter aimed "to present the clothes of the present day" (Roche, 1994: 476).

The first true fashion magazine?

In the 1770s a new standard was reached for fashion illustration with the publication of *La Gallerie des Modes*. The next famous French fashion magazine was published under three titles: between 1785 and 1786 as *Le Cabinet des Modes,* then *Le Magazine des Modes Nouvelles Françaises et Anglaises* until 1789, and finally between 1790 and 1793 as *Le Journal de la Mode et du Goût.* As pointed out elsewhere (Miller in Bartlett, Cole and Rocamora, 2013), La galerie des modes consisted of albums with colored engravings published on a regular basis between 1778 and 1779 by Jean Esnauts and Michel Rapilly under the formidable title *La Gallerie des modes et des costumes français dessinés d'après nature. Gravés par les plus Célèbres Artistes en ce genre et colorés avec le plus gran soin par Madame Le Beau.*

Ouvrage commence en l'anné 1778. A Paris, chez les S.rs Esnauts et Rapilly, rue St. Jacques, à la Ville de Coutances. Avec Priv. Du roi (Morini, 2006: 29). James Laver considered this album as a "pioneer in the field of the fashion plate," and he references the distinction made by Vyvyan Holland (second son of Oscar Wilde) in his *Hand-coloured Fashion Plates, 1770–1899* between what he called the "fashion plate" and the "costume plate," with the latter representing clothes "after the event," such as Wenceslas Hollar in his *Ornatus Muliebirs Anglicanus*, published in 1640, or the work that Jean Dieu de Saint-Jean did in France in his admirable engravings of male and female costume at the Court of Louis XIV (Laver, 1969: 145–6) (Figure 4.5). Patriotically perhaps, Laver considered that the "first true fashion plates" were not French but rather English as published in *The Lady's Magazine* from 1770 onward. There were also important seventeenth-century precedents that depicted ladies and beauties of the court after great masters and with verses and descriptions appended (Figure 4.6). He would also have known about the finely detailed engravings of women's fashions that were included in the pocket-books or almanacs of ladies from the 1750s (Figure 4.7). What made the new type of fashion prints so special was their immediacy: they really told of the latest "must have" fashions (Figure 4.8). And they certainly did not depict made-up fashions, as the recent research of Johannes Pietsch on the *Gallerie des Modes* and Bissonette on the *Journal des Dames* has proven (Pietsch; Bissonette, 2015).

The first fashion magazine: *Le Cabinet des Modes*

The founder of the magazine was Jean Antoine Brun (aka Le Brun Tossa), and its first issue was published in 1785 under the full title *Cabinet des Modes, ou des Modes Nouvelles*. What is even more interesting is the extended subtitle that captures its very clear aims and objectives as well as its content, including the charming specification "described in a clear manner." This is continued with by the lengthy

> and represented by plates and illuminated etchings. Magazine which gives an exact and prompt knowledge of clothes and finery of the persons of the one and the other sex, also of new furniture of all kinds, of new decorations, home embellishments, the latest shapes of carriages, silversmithing and generally all that fashion offers as singular, agreeable or interesting in every genre.

At the bottom of the page information about the magazine is also added: "This magazine consists of twenty four issues per year and is published every fifteen days. Every issue consists of eight pages *in octavo* and three illuminated etching." The success of the magazine was instantaneous because of its popular formula:

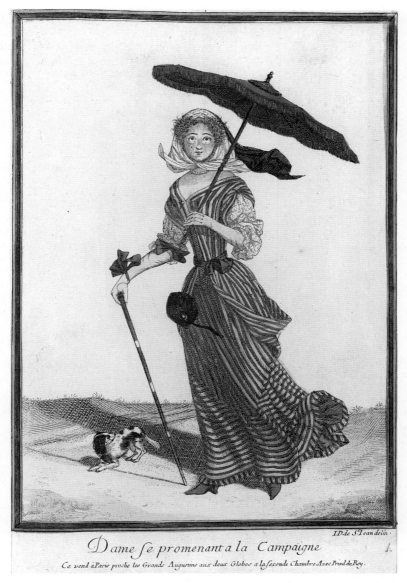

Dame ſe promenant a la Campaigne

Ce vend à Paris proche les Grands Augustins aux deux Globes a la ſeconde Chambre Avec Priv du Roy.

I.D. de S. Iean delin.

FIGURE 4.5 *Jean Dieu de Saint-Jean (active 1675–1695),* Dame se promenant a la Campaigne, *in "Recueil des modes de la cour de France," Paris, 1675–7, hand-colored engraving on paper. Sheet: 14 3/8 × 9 3/8 in. (36.51 × 23.81 cm); composition: 11 3/8 × 7 5/8 in. (28.89 × 19.37 cm). Los Angeles County Museum of Art. Purchased with funds provided by The Eli and Edythe L. Broad Foundation, Mr. and Mrs. H. Tony Oppenheimer, Mr. and Mrs. Reed Oppenheimer, Hal Oppenheimer, Alice and Nahum Lainer, Mr. and Mrs. Gerald Oppenheimer, Ricki and Marvin Ring, Mr. and Mrs. David Sydorick, the Costume Council Fund, and members of the Costume Council (M.2002.57.50).*

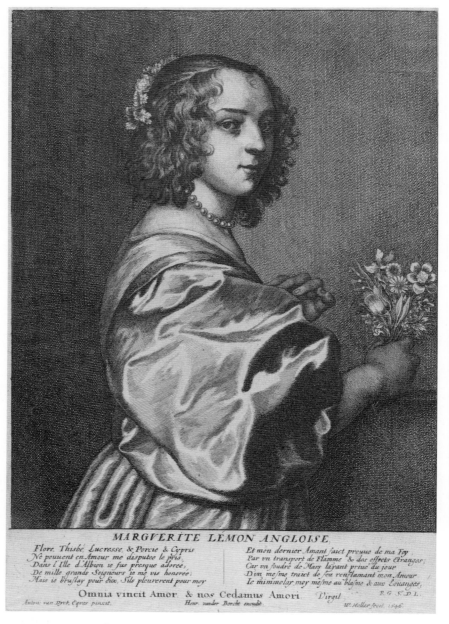

FIGURE 4.6 *Anthony van Dyck, artist; W. Hollar, engraver: "Margeurite Lemon Angloise," 1646, engraving. Courtesy Lewis Walpole Library Yale University.*

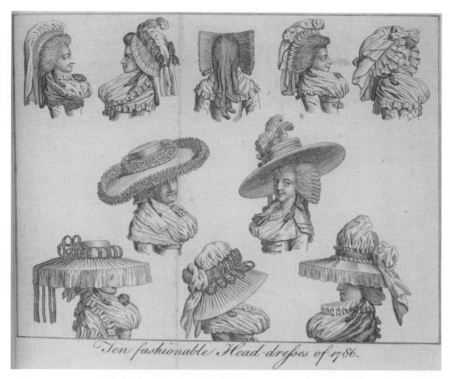

Ten fashionable Head-dresses of 1786.

FIGURE 4.7 *"Ten Fashionable Head-dresses of 1786," a folding page from a printed pocketbook, England, one of an assembled album of 238 depictions of hairstyles and hats in 28 pages, 1777–99, England. Photograph © Cora Ginsburg/ Titi Halle, New York.*

> *Le Cabinet des modes*, among others found a formula whose immediate success justified both its policy and its investment; it accepted the role of intermediary between those who received and those who created the consumer revolution in clothes as in other things, and this placed the press in the slipstream of fashion. (Roche, 1994: 482)

The images in the journals were used in all sorts of manners by readers and consumers, including even cutting them up to make a category of objects that museums and collectors called "dressed prints", which implied the addition of glued sand, lichens, and textiles to the print. Alternatively, the print itself might be cut out and have inserted in it or on it fine textiles and braid from behind. This tradition of amending prints and adding "textile information" and effects was particularly prominent in seventeenth and eighteenth prints of the Saints, who were equally beautifully dressed in the Catholic Church in real textiles, often of early dates. It is a good example of how longer traditions inform what might seem like new practices.

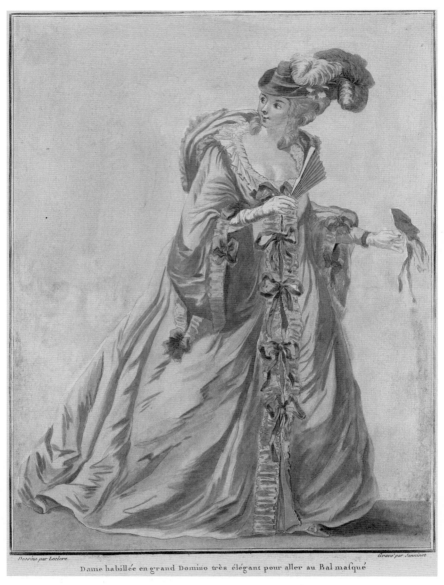

Dame habillée en grand Domino très élégant pour aller au Bal masqué

FIGURE 4.8 *Pierre-Thomas LeClerc, draughtsman; Janinet, engraver; Esnauts et Rapilly, publisher, "Gallerie des Modes et Costumes Français". 39e Cahier (bis) des Costumes Français, 34e Suite d'Habillemens les plus à la mode. 252(bis) Dame habillée en grand Domino ... 1783, Paris, hand-colored engraving on laid paper 41.6 × 27.0 cm (16 3/8 × 10 5/8 in.) Copyright The Museum of Fine Arts Boston, The Elizabeth Day McCormick Collection 2017.*

So what was new about the *Cabinet des Modes*? This may be construed as stating the obvious, because what else can a publication starting with the most modest, such as the *corantos,* do but communicate? Roche goes on to elaborate about the special identity of the journalists who perfected so successful a formula in the fashion periodical. Given that no such thing as a professional journalist—never mind fashion journalists—existed during the eighteenth century, their achievement is even more remarkable. Thus, the first fashion journalists, or rather the first journalists who paid attention to fashion, came from the literary tradition. There is nothing new here given that it was only in the 1970s when the first degrees in journalism in the UK were founded, including the *Cardiff School of Journalism Media and Cultural Studies* (from 1970 at Cardiff University) and the internationally renowned *Department of Journalism* at the City University in London (from 1976). Until that time, the majority of the journalists working in the industry came from the humanities, e.g., literature, history, or philosophy, and they were trained "on the job" in the time-honored manner of the medieval professional guilds.

But how was this to be achieved? As Roche observed, by progressing on three fronts:

- it had to discover men and women capable of achieving recognition and continued success, among them powerful personages in possession of the literary field
- it had to seek out its public
- it had to widen its appeal by offering both a new type of subject and new methods (Roche, 1994: 482–3)

In the second version of the *Cabinet des Modes*—*Le Magazine des Modes Nouvelles Françaises et Anglaises*—we note that French fashion was paralleled with English fashion, which meant that they accepted it as equal or at least complementary. One of the reasons was that the French *rococo* style was becoming too extravagant even for Versailles and the restrained English "look" influenced by country life was adopted by the French aristocracy, who also embraced a new pure form of "neo-classicism." The magazine continued to be published under its third title until 1793, but what is remarkable is that a fashion magazine was even published during the bloodiest revolution in modern history.

The fashion magazine as "mirror" of its time

Fashion often reflects on its own past. Its history was often written by journalists and scavans, who would now be considered amateurs. They often provided insightful overviews very probably influenced by reading older texts and perusing images that they themselves took an interest in. There was even a category of writing called "it narratives" in the eighteenth century, in which articles of clothing were personified and allowed to speak, often going on amusing and even wicked journeys through the streets (Christina Lupton (ed.), *British It-Narratives, 1750–1830. Volume 3: Clothes and Transportation* (London: Pickering & Chatto, 2012)) (Figure 4.9). Novelists, too, found the resonance of the images from old fashion periodicals evocative. The fashion plates of the eighteenth century were already iconic by the 1830s. To underscore provincialism, a scene in Gustave Flaubert's *Madame Bovary, Provincial Lives* (trans. and with intro. by Geoffrey Wall, preface Michèle Roberts, Penguin Classics, London, 2003) described a shop in a village thus:

> when it was windy you could hear the creaking of the set of little copper basins hanging from their rods, which did duty as the sign of the wig-maker's shop. By way of decoration, it had an ancient fashion-plate stuck on one of the window-panes and a wax bust of a woman, which had yellow hair. (Bovary 60)

Such periodicals and engravings would have been quite common on secondhand and junk stalls in the first half of the twentieth century—or were thrown into the tip—whereas in the period from the 1970s, they rose in value and museums around the world began to collect and highlight them as important parts of their holdings (Robyn Healy, "Fashion and Textiles Collection," *Art & Australia. Australian National Gallery Special Number*, 20: 1, Spring 1982, 98–101). An historical overview of the emergence of the fashion magazine was written by the poet Henri Bidou in the introduction of the first issue of the luxury fashion periodical *Gazette du bon ton* and published in its November 1912 issue. Bidou argued that the first proper fashion magazine in the modern sense of the word was Le Brun Tossa's *Le Cabinet des Modes,* which included "plates after Desrais et Deframe, philosophical varieties, anecdotes, literary productions, comparisons between French and English fashions, which extended also to Jewellery and furniture" (Bidou in Miller: Bartlett, Cole, Rocamora, 2013: 18–19).

But there was another function that Le Brun Tossa's magazines fulfilled, and on this occasion they really did become mirrors of their time, charted in the changes noticeable not only in what people wore but all the other aspects listed by *Le Cabinet des Modes.* We notice this particularly with fashion which altered from the opulence of the rococo to a sober post-revolutionary style imposed by the Jacobin "reign of terror." The Cabinet has saved for posterity many of the startling fashions worn during the period of Revolution.

Between 1793 and 1797 all magazines were silenced by the Jacobin terror, only to return during the Directory period, when the *Journal des Dames et des Modes* reigned supreme in terms of influence (Ribeiro, 1988: 21–2). Little wonder given the unique—at times even humorous, albeit of the black variety—manner they chose to report the gruesome events such as the "bals des victimes" at which some dancers wore their hair cropped "à la victime" and others ribbons like the cut of the blade across their necks.

(1)

MEMOIRS

AND INTERESTING

ADVENTURES

OF AN

Embroidered WAISTCOAT.

 HE Succefs of a late Pamphlet of my writing, having put a little Money in my Pocket, I confidered the different Situation of the Mind, in Circumftances of Eafe, from thofe of Depreffion and Want, I

B   found

FIGURE 4.9 *"Memoirs and Interesting Adventures of an Embroidered Waistcoat",* *frontispiece, London, J. Brooks, 1760. Courtesy Lewis Walpole Library, Yale University.*

Although Germany and its myriad publications are less well known in the English-speaking world, early fashion magazines were also published there during the Enlightenment. Young publisher Friederich Justin Bertuch announced in 1785 the publication of the magazine *Journal des Luxus und der Moden* (published until 1827). This was the first German magazine dedicated exclusively to fashion, "filled with boastful self-confidence" regarding the quality of the authors and the fineness of the consumer goods (Purdy in Riello and McNeil, 2010: 238).

In 1829, the novelist and budding fashion historian Caroline de la Motte Fouqué (1773–1831) wrote a series of articles about fashion, four of which were published as *Geschichte der* Moden *1785–1829* in *Journal des Luxus und der Moden,* complemented by a selection of plates dated between 1786 and 1827 and an epilogue written by Dorothea Böck (Union Verlag Berlin, Democratic Republic of Germany, 1987).

What makes these plates special is—given that Germany did not have a bloody revolution—the fact that the *Journal des Luxus und der Moden* was in a position to document the transition for the Rococo to the neo-classical style of the early nineteenth century, not only in fashion, but also furniture and accessories, much like its French counterparts which could not—for the obvious reasons—provide the same continuity.

La vie Parisienne *(1863–1970) as mirror of its time*

By the nineteenth century the fashion magazine was an established institution, catering for an exigent readership, and the consequence was that they transcended the remit of clothes to spill into other areas of general interest. Fashion magazines joined the numerous other genres of writing that the avid women readers of the nineteenth century embraced, from novels to histories to periodicals (Figure 4.10). Lithography made colored illustrations much cheaper (Figure 4.11), although the cheapest publications remained in black and white until the beginning of the twentieth century. Women were often addressed explicitly by the press (Figure 4.12) and were catered to by a burgeoning number of fashion and "shelter" or home living magazines, including specialist North American numbers (Figure 4.13).

Thus, the weekly *La vie Parisienne* founded in 1863 by Emil Marcelin (1825–1887) included—apart from the obligatory fashion reporting— "stories, news, sports, theatre, music and the arts." Marcelin enlisted also the collaboration of some of the finest writers so that the list of contributors read more like the "who's who" of nineteenth-century Paris intelligentsia (Miller in: Bartlett, Cole, and Rocamora, 2013: 20). Thus, in the issue dated Saturday, January 4, 1913, published fifty years after its inauguration in 1863, we find an article entitled "Le cinquatenaire de L V P" signed by Charles Saglio, celebrating its success:

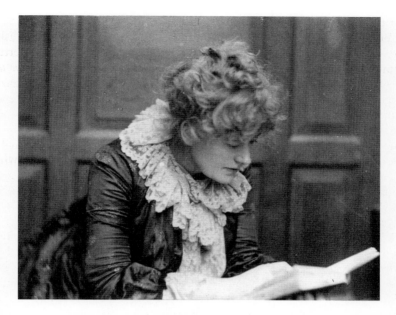

FIGURE 4.10 *Frederick Hollyer, Ellen Terry;* Portraits of many persons of note photographed by Frederick Hollyer in three volumes, *vol. III, 1886, platinum print. Given by Eleanor M. Hollyer 1938. Victoria and Albert Museum 7861–1938.* © *Victoria and Albert Museum, London.*

Ellen Terry, famous late-nineteenth-century British actress, is shown here in a graceful act of reading, probably a history or Shakespeare.

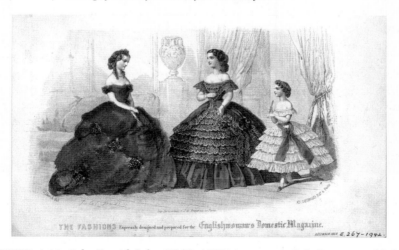

FIGURE 4.11 *Jules David, Jules (1808–1892) (engraver); S.O. Beeton (publisher), Lamoureux & J. De Beauvais, Paris (printer), "The Fashions, expressly designed and prepared for the Englishwoman's Domestic Magazine, December 1860," lithograph, colored by hand, ink, and watercolor on paper. Victoria and Albert Museum. Given by Mr. A. R. Harvey, E.267-1942.* © *Victoria and Albert Museum, London.*

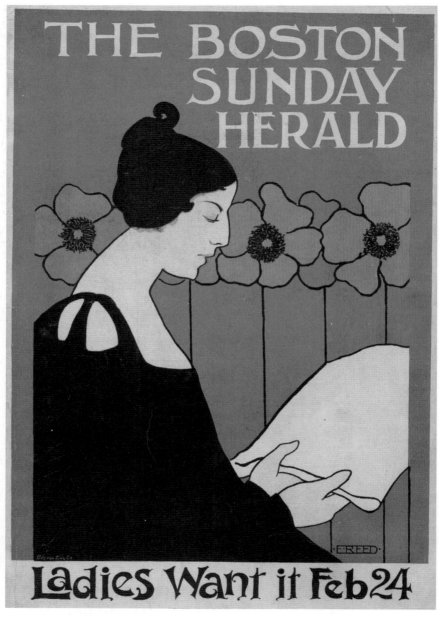

FIGURE 4.12 *Ethel Reed, "The Boston Sunday Herald—ladies want it", February 24, 1895 or 1901[?], Boston MA Eng. Co., color lithograph, 43.7 × 30.1 cm. Courtesy of the Library of Congress Prints and Photographs Division, Washington, D.C., POS—US.R44, no. 3 (B size) [P&P].*
  Possibly a self-portrait by the artist.

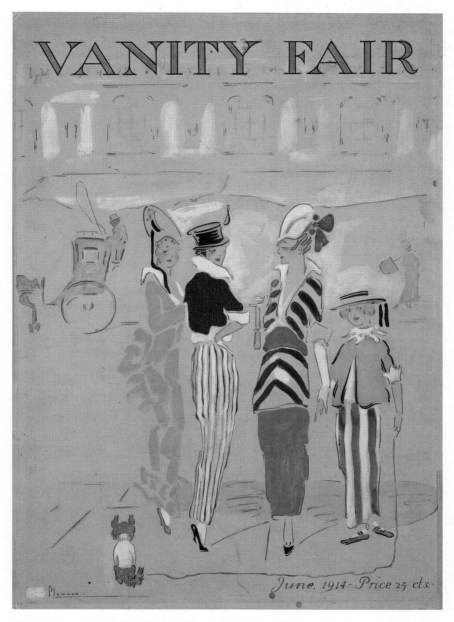

FIGURE 4.13 *Ethel M'Clellan Plummer (1888–1936), Vanity Fair on the Avenue, June 1914, cover drawing, India ink, gouache, and watercolor over pencil, 44.2 × 30.4 cm (sheet). Courtesy of the Library of Congress Prints and Photographs Division, Washington, D.C., SWANN—no. 1272 (B size) [P&P].*

The 4 of January 1863, today we celebrate exactly half a century from the date of the publication of the first issue of *La Vie Parisienne* whose success, since it was first published is by now well known. This elegant and spiritual journal has been depicting on a daily basis an apparently frivolous but in fact profoundly true and sincere picture of Parisian fashionable life.

The author introduces with wit and charm some of its contributors as follows:

From the beginning, here are some of the most assiduous collaborators of our magazine: here is Taine with his sparkling notes on Paris, here is Edmond About, Charles Baudelaire, Champfleury, Charles Monselet, Quatrelles, (the pseudonym of Ernest L'Epiné), Henry Maret, Francisque Sarcey and the spiritual marquis de Massa. (Saglio, 1913–14)

But its prime function was to present "a true and sincere picture of Parisian fashionable life," and in this sense it reviews Charles Baudelaire's definition of modernity (*modernité*) from one of his salon better known as "*The Painter of Modern Life.*" First published in 1863 and dedicated to the painter Constantin Guys whom Baudelaire considered to be that painter of modern life, modernity was defined as "the transient, the fleeting, the contingent; it is one half of art, the other being the eternal and the immovable" (Baudelaire, 1972: 401).

Existing statistics confirm that if we compare the number of fashion magazines published during the eighteenth century with subsequent centuries, we see their numbers increase exponentially and that can only mean one thing: increasing demand. We find this confirmation in Hilaire and Meyer Hiler's list of periodicals published in 1939: *Bibliography of Costume: A dictionary Catalogue of about Eight Thousand Books and Periodicals* (The H.W. Wilson Co, N.Y., 1939). During the eighteenth century the market was dominated by French magazines, but the situation changed during the nineteenth century when it becomes international by including English and American magazines. The list of French magazines contains some of their finest publications starting with *La vie Parisienne*— already mentioned—*La Mode Illustrée* (first published in 1860), *Art et la Mode de L'Élégance* (first published 1881); for England, we have *The Tailor and Cutter* (first published 1866) and *The Young Ladies Journal* (first published 1864); and for the US, *Harper's Bazaar* (first published 1867) and *Vogue* (incorporating *Vanity Fair*, first published 1892). For the twentieth-century pride of place went to the French magazines *Femina* (first published in 1901) and *L'Élégance Feminine* (first published in 1933).

The twentieth century: New departures for the fashion magazine

Case study: *Madame*—Exploring social issues

Charles Saglio was right regarding the role fashion magazines played on the cultural scene at a level which transcended frivolity, although this was often achieved by emulating just such an approach. An important role fashion magazines assumed during the twentieth century was their coverage of issues not directly related to fashion, in itself a new *métier*.

Fashion writing was still in a process of transition: from a descriptive approach which paralleled the visual image of the garment, to analysis and criticism made possible by the founding of the *maisons de couture* inaugurated by Charles Frederick Worth during the second half of the nineteenth century.

Moreover, a multitude of new interests—science and technology, the body beautiful (cosmetics), fashion, the theatre, and the other visual arts, but above all a special interest in social issues—were now being addressed.

Regarding the latter, we find examples in the pages of the English magazine *Madame* (1895–1913). Thus, in the Saturday, February 3, 1906, issue we find a report from Paris by Jeanne Vinniers entitled "A reportage—impressionistic (sic) about what fashionable *parisiennes* wear!" The approach was still descriptive but we learn about something new, the process of illustration: the outfits selected for the magazine were sketched in situ by the magazine illustrator. Thus, we find just such a reportage in *Madame* (February 3, 1906):

> For the evening and on some—not all—women Josephine robes are lovely, and I had a little sketch made last Monday night in the foyer at the Opera of one that seemed to me eminently desirable. The material was hand-painted gauze, bold branches of mauve glycine meandering over a background of palest grey-blue and on the hem of the skirt, also on the bodice there were the loveliest medallions of black Chantilly with centres of mauve velvet embroidered in gold. (*Madame*, Saturday, February 3, 1906: 214)

But this was about to change with the proliferation of *maisons de couture* in Paris: instead of making quick sketches of the latest fashion worn at occasions such as the opera, the fashion journalist visited the fashion houses and reported on the latest collections, and this is how real fashion criticism made its entrance. *Madame* provided a regular column entitled "Professions for Women" signed "Helena," offering advice regarding the job market, especially the "Civil Service," for which we find a tempting advertisement regarding the benefits on offer, and in the issue dated January 27, 1906, they are listed as "generous holiday, moderate hours, a reasonable chance for a rise, and a wedding present on resignement [sic] for marriage, inducements that every profession does not offer to women." The four specific positions on offer for which there was an open competition were girl clerks, women clerks, female learners, and female sorters. Age was very important: the "age of application must be between 16 and 18"; "between the ages of 18 and 20 they were eligible"; and "the girl must be between 15 and 18." The clerical positions on offer were mostly for the Post Office and the Savings Bank Department: "and one of the sinecures of the Civil Service is the position of superintendent in the Savings Bank which brings a salary of £320 to £500 and the latter's assistant £200 a year" (*Madame*, January 27, 1906: 230). The journalist assigned to so specific a job was signed with the pseudonym "Helene," which is significant because in a world still dominated by male journalists, the choice of a woman was deliberate in order to reassure women readers of her credentials.

The body beautiful: Science and technology

We have a charming example which combines humor with the latest developments in the field of cosmetics in a lighthearted manner proving that although fashion magazines may have appeared frivolous, they were in fact—as Charles Saglio rightly pointed out in *La vie Parisienne*—an accurate mirror of their times. Thus, in the August 1913 issue of the *Gazette du bon ton*, we find a funny article illustrated by none other than Paul Poiret's illustrator Georges Lepape, about a new practice coming from England: **eyebrow plucking**. In this article, its author signing under the pseudonym *Galaor* was "deploring" the latest attempt adopted by fashion-conscious women to "correct nature" through this horrendous new practice that Galaor considered to be a "barbaric attack" on the eyebrows. Moreover, he lamented, Buffon (an eighteenth-century naturalist) in his *Histoire Naturelle* (page 288, volume IV) regarded eyebrows the most important element after the eyes, of the human physiognomy. And then, Galaor continued, the "genial *inventeur anglais*" suddenly decided "*corrigeons la Nature!*" and opened an "*atelier-laboratoire*," and Galaor even provided a description of the aforesaid practice:

> With the patience of a Danaide, and the most minute instruments this man removes the misplaced eyebrows with "*une mystérieuse matière*" whose secret he does not reveal, and then paints on the nude face new eyebrows in the exact place where they should have been and thus "even the most exigent" of women can realize her ideal of beauty. His invention so appealed to women that they were flocking in droves to England, willingly submitting themselves to this "torture" at the hands of its "awful executioner." (*Gazette du bon ton*, nr. August 10, 1913: 305–8).

In the February 1937 issue of *L'Officiel de la Couture de la Mode de Paris*, we find an article about the *scientific* advances of cosmetic surgery by a Dr. Dantrelle, entitled *"La Chirurgie des Rides"* (surgery for wrinkles). His "scientific explanation" referred to a new medical intervention—"lifting"—on which Dr. Dantrelle commented, and this is very interesting, "should not be reserved only for women of an advanced age but offered in a preventive manner to younger women." The conclusion was that while "la chirurgie des rides" (surgery of the wrinkles) had a period "de tâtonnement" (trial and error) at present, it has become "the most certain, the most inoffensive and the best method science has on offer in the service of beauty." A "lifting" well executed, according to this story, deletes the wrinkles and folds around the mouth and the accentuated double chin, and renders the face unified, smooth, and considerably rejuvenated, but its greatest merit is to have reconstituted the oval shape of the face (*L'Officiel de la Couture de la Mode de Paris*, February 1937: 85). It may come as a surprise to the twenty-first-century reader that the claims made by the cosmetic industry are by no means of recent date, and we find an uncanny parallel between the claims made by botulinum toxic injections (better known as *Botox*) to eliminate the wrinkles and folds of the face and return to it the smooth appearance of youth and those of Dr. Dantrelle in the February 1937 issue of *L'Officiel*.

Hardly qualifying as cosmetic surgery, it becomes obvious that these were rather benign practices by comparison with contemporary practices such as tattooing, body piercing, and scarification to extreme forms of surgery exemplified by the French artist Orlan "on behalf of art," and we can conclude that the relationship between "the body beautiful" (cosmetics) and fashion has changed beyond recognition.

Culture and the arts

A seminal aspect of the fashion magazine was the professionalism with which they covered myriad cultural and artistic events: music, theatre, literature, and the visual arts were all were given extensive coverage by established writers and critics. To return to *La vie Parisienne*, in the October 5, 1912, issue we find a review signed by their columnist, *Doricas*, covering the most exciting avant-garde institution in Paris: the *Salon d'Automne*—already reviewed in *L'Intransigeant* by none other than the influential critic Guillaume Apollinaire—where he commented that its chief attraction was "the decorative arts group," but he could not say more because "our friends are not ready" (Apollinaire in Motherwell (ed), 1972: 17–18). "Doricas" had no such reservations and she provided a lighthearted analysis of the new presence of the decorative arts at a salon hitherto dedicated to the fine arts:

Ah, *"mon enfant!"* what rest! in this room they built a town: on one side, the house of a rich *entrepreneur*, all spangled with roses carved in wood by Süe, on the other side a cubist mansion, yes, cubist, whose architect is called Duchamp-Villon, in which is housed a whole phalanstery: Richard Desvallières forged the iron, André Marc made the furniture, Marie Laurencin the overmantel etc. and to be perfectly honest this is not bad at all! (*La vie Parisienne*, Saturday, January 6, 1912: 713–16)

The magazine ran also an amusing column entitled "On dit ... on dit"—translated here by us as "Tit bits"—whose lighthearted tenor was meant for entertainment and no doubt the joy of gossiping. Thus, in the October 26, 1913, issue we find a reference to the Futurists and to the philosopher who inspired them: Henri Bergson, here patriotically, but mistakenly credited to be "inventor of the unconscious," an understandable error given that the writings of Sigmund Freud, although well known in professional circles, were not common knowledge. The piece was entitled "Le philosophe futuriste," and in it the anonymous writer starts by lamenting that these poor futurists do not enjoy good press and they were even reproached for being foreigners (all five Futurists who founded the movement were Italians). But the Futurists appeared to have found themselves a defender, who was none other than "M. Bergson, our grand *philosophe*, the inventor of the '*subconscient*'" (subconscious).

The writer goes on to comment on M. Bergson's passion for Futurism which explained his presence at all the openings of their exhibitions. But that was not all: M. Bergson "even owns" in his "*petite maison de Neuilly,*" "deux tableaux du 'Fauvisme' le plus intransigeant" (*La vie Parisienne*, October 26, 1912: 76). But even if the little paintings he owned were not Futurist but Fauvist (we forgive the author for such a confusion), M. Bergson certainly appreciated avant-garde art.

A more serious approach can be found in the bi-monthly *Vogue* (the American edition dated August 1, 1916) in an analysis of John Singer Sargent's infamous portrait of "Mme. X" that had just been acquired by the Metropolitan Museum of Art in New York:

> The subject is Mme. Gautereau, a redoubtable Parisian beauty of the early eighties. Mme. Gautereau however refused to accept it, giving as a reason for her refusal that Sargent had pitched in somewhat too frank a vein. The painter did not insist on her carrying out her side of the contract and promptly and obligingly created another portrait of her ... Sargent decided however to send the rejected canvas to the Paris Salon of 1884 (the year of the painting) where, under the designation of "Portrait of Mme. G" it made an immediate success. (*Vogue*, August 1, 1916, p.72)

In another reportage for *Vogue* (the American edition, dated January 15, 1922) signed Mary Fanton-Roberts, entitled "Ultra-Modern French Art in New York," Ms Fanton-Roberts reported on an exhibition held at the Wanamaker gallery: "we have to refresh our memories a little to realize fully that France also leads the world in Art and Fashion," and she offered a perceptive overview of the Parisian art world:

> There are no preconceived ideas of art in France: tradition, memories, yes, but no halos for the past and no barriers for the future. Since the war, art lovers waited and wondered about post-war French art.

The two female artists singled out by Fanton-Roberts were the fashionable beauty Irène Lagut and the art deco painter Marie Laurencin. Fanton-Roberts's critical comments about the latter's paintings can only be considered as outstanding: "The work of Marie Laurencin indicates a tendency in modern French art towards a certain, cruel, graceful decadence." The journalist selected two examples of her work, one being a portrait of the wife of the critic André Salmon, harshly summed up as follows:

> Marie Laurencin's portrait of Mme. André Salmon is a painting of a woman who reminds one somewhat of Mme. Bovary, sullen, self centred again with a narrow jaw and the eyes greedy for sensation. There is sadness but rather the sadness of an unsatisfied woman, one carrying tragic memories. It is a painting of the bitter acceptance of life, ruthlessly seeking compensation. The colour is presented in interesting masses ... the gown blue and rose, the background rose and grey. The effect ... is, as a whole, decorative in form and colour, without depth, without body in the drawing.

Fanton-Roberts was equally ungenerous—but on this occasion with good justification—of Lagut's work: "Irène Lagut is more definitely decorative and much less direct and human" (*Vogue*, January 15, 1922, p. 50; continued on p. 80).

Fanton-Roberts's critical comments are as impressive as those of her better-known male contemporary critics, and if the snooty art historians would have taken the trouble to consult fashion magazines regarded as "lightweight," they would have discovered a treasure-trove of original criticism and research regarding the relationship of fashion and the visual arts.

Fashion and the stage

The relationship between *haute couture* and the stage and that between theatrical costume and fashion is an important dimension covered in fashion magazines from both perspectives: the influence of fashion on the theatre and that of the theatre on fashion. Thus, the critic of the *Gazette du bon ton*, Lise-Léon Bloom in her column entitled "Le goût au théâtre" categorically stated (February 1913: 149–52) that fashion is inspired by theatrical costume and not the other way round: *le théâtre precède la mode.*

In the March 1913 issue of the same magazine, we find an article signed by Gabriel Mourey entitled "Les robes de Bakst," whose humorous opening paragraph tells us that the dresses designed by Bakst have taken over the salons, the artists' ateliers, the tea houses, the train carriages; in fact, "partout" (everywhere), the one and only subject of debate being "the dresses designed by Bakst and crafted by Mme. Paquin et M. Joire" (*Gazette du bon ton*, March: 162). In the same issue, Lise-Léon Blum gives several examples, among them the relationship between the actress Andrée Megard she referred to as "Mme. Megard" and the house of Redfern. Before embarking to play Roxane in Edmund de Rostand's *Cyrano de Bergerac*, she approached her "couturier habituel," and the result was a perfect symbiosis which "Mme. Megard and M. Redefern have created." Another example was that of a *couturier* working for the theatre, and that *couturier* was none other than Paul Poiret. He designed the costumes for a play by Jacques Ricepin entitled *Harem* in which the main part was played by Ricepin's wife Cora Lapracerie. The play was premiered at the *Théâtre de la Renaissance* in Paris on March 20, 1913, and the theatre critic had this to say:

> But if the costumes were inspired from Persian miniatures and Japanese prints it is with a modern interpretation, in fact with a violently modern interpretation with which he shocked with his excess of novelty rather the use of archaism or exoticism … They are attired in swaying tunics boned to hold out the skirt which looks like a lamp shade over hobble skirts … Every material under the sky was used: pearls, fur, gauze, brocade, and even textiles woven in metal which gave M. Jean Worms the appearance of a lacquer prince. (*Gazette du bon ton*, March 1913: 188)

The review finishes with a witty comment regarding Denise's (Paul Poiret's wife and muse) presence in the auditorium "dressed as if ready to step onto the stage, with a heavy silver helmet covering her hair completed by an incredible bunch of black feathers placed in the centre" (*Gazette du bon ton*, March 1913). Such theatrical fashions can be seen in an ensemble retailed by Poiret at the American store Gimbels (Figure 4.14). Women had not looked so bizarre since the 1790s (the period of the Directoire immediately following the Revolution), and it seems that the fashions were set in this immediate pre-World War I period by the stage rather than by politics.

The changing face of the fashion magazine: Case study—*Harper's Bazaar*

The first American fashion magazine published in 1867 became also one of the most influential. Its subtitle "A Repository of Fashion, Pleasure and Instruction" tells the reader of its remit which combined pleasure with instruction, but above all it was reporting on the latest fashions. Initially

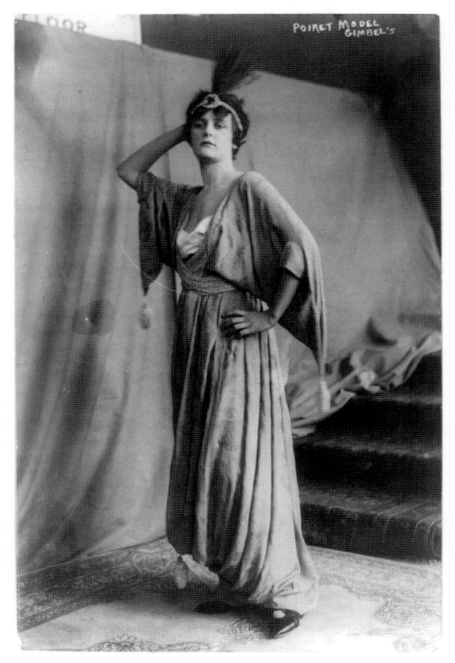

FIGURE 4.14 *Poiret model—Gimbels, March 1914, photographic print. Photo by Bain News Service. Courtesy of the Library of Congress Prints and Photographs Division, Washington, D.C. LC-USZ62-85524 (b&w film copy neg.).*

a weekly at ten cents a copy, *Harper's Bazaar* quickly became a trend-setter, and considering its venerable age, its formula was a successful one. Moreover, comparison between issues published during the nineteenth, the twentieth, and the twenty-first centuries reveal another winning formula: the magazine's ability to move with the times.

The nineteenth century—Harper's Bazaar: *1891*

If we peruse the issues published in 1891, the main focus was on the latest fashions, but we find also features. It is important to note that its editorial policies were informed by a common denominator: its readers were women! Thus, in the Saturday July 4, 1891, issue we have a fashion article entitled "Summer Gowns," whose approach was entirely descriptive paralleling the illustration provided. Roland Barthes famously argued in *The Fashion System* (first published in 1967) that **written clothing** and **visual image clothing** do the same job, and this is the case in the above example. Therefore, the written text and visual image in *Harper's Bazaar* should fulfill the same function, but in fact they do not!

> I open a fashion magazine; I see that two different garments are being dealt with here. The first is the one presented to me as photographed or drawn—it is image-clothing. The second is the same garment, but described, transformed into language; this dress photographed on the right, becomes on the left: *a leather belt, with a rose stuck in it, worn above the waist, on a soft Shetland dress*; this is the written garment ... the first structure is plastic, the second verbal. (Barthes, 1990: 3)

In our 1891 example, the magazine provides an image and a written text, both referencing a third term introduced by Barthes: the **technological object**—a pretty summer gown.

> Wisteria coloured flowered lawn is the material of a pretty summer gown illustrated. It is made over plain lawn of the same shade. A gathered flounce with a heading is at the foot of the shirt around the front and sides. The pointed bodice is cut down at the throat and is trimmed at the edges of the front with a lavender ribbon and a jabot of white lace. The lace and ribbon trimming descends in a point at the back. The elbow sleeves are puffed with a ribbon. (*Harper's Bazaar*, Saturday, July 1891: 513)

What the text adds to the image are details such as the materials used, e.g., "lawn" or in Barthes's text "Shetland dress," which is also "soft." But even if the textile specialist identifies Shetland wool as distinct from other wools because of its "softness," the use of the adjective adds something to the way we relate to the dress; but we can ponder how would a fashion image convey this sense of "softness"? The answer is that the image cannot do this job alone, and while our pleasure in admiring the visual image is unmediated by language, the use of "softness" in the written text is mediated through the intellect and we therefore may even use "softness" as an evaluative term: softness may also be about loveliness and tactile pleasure.

In the same issue we find a feature by Elizabeth Eliott entitled "The Heroine's Gowns" in which Barthes's aforementioned distinction can also be used: thus read in the opening rather Proustian paragraph:

> Through countless pages in all tongues and times the heroine goes. Serene and stately, saucy and piquante, gentle and loving, or fierce and fiery, whatever her role may be in the drama, she is always costumed to suit it and like the visible heroines who appear before us on the stage, we often remember the toilette when we forget the wearer. (p. 513)

Interestingly, the author makes the point that the writer must put before the reader a picture **in writing** that should be as good as "Sir Joshua Reynolds's portrait of the Duchess of Devonshire with his brush," because in order to make the portrait clear "one must see her costume; for to a woman her clothes are only second in importance to her soul's salvation and not always to that." As a case study Elizabeth Eliott chose none other than Jane Austen:

> Miss Austen among all the multifarious details of "Pride and Prejudice," "Sense and Sensibility" and other alliterative Romances which our ancestors had time to read, dwells very little upon the attire of her Elizabeths and Carolines. The face, figure and carriage of these young ladies is minutely portrayed, indeed they go so far as to have "deportment"—a quality quite unknown to the modern heroine. The amount of fortune they may expect from their parents is usually stated also with gratifying precision but the author scorns such frivolities as clothes except for the most casual mention. (*Harper's Bazaar*, Saturday, July 1891)

But then the author comments times have changed and instead of ignoring attire, writers dwell on it with "a lavish extravagance":

> Whether the occasion requires the dainty and piquant costume or the sumptuous and elegant, the heroine always has it, regardless of expense. (*Harper's Bazaar*, Saturday, July 1891)

The example chosen is that of Daisy Miller, the heroine of a novella written by Henry James in 1878. Its heroine, a wealthy American *nouveau riche* young lady arrives at a fashionable resort in Switzerland, where she upsets

society with her carefree attitude interpreted as reckless, and unlike Jane
Austen, Henry James relishes in describing her lavish costumes:

> Daisy Miller wore white muslin when she stepped down the gravel
> path across Winterbourne's horizon, but it was a "white muslin with
> a hundred frills and flounces and knots of pale-coloured ribbon" and
> "she carried a white parasol with a deep border of embroidery" and Mr.
> James adds, as a finishing touch to the picture, that she was "strikingly,
> admirably, pretty." James always gives one the idea that he could go
> into any minutiae of detail about toilette if he chose. (*Harper's Bazaar*,
> Saturday, July 1891)

The twentieth century: Harper's Bazaar, *1952*

If we move fast forward to the 1950s the balance is tilted toward visuals, not
illustrations, but a new dimension conspicuously absent in the 1891 issue:
illustrated advertising is added. Thus, in the March 1952 issue, pages 1–124
are devoted to advertising. How things are changing! But the magazine was
proud of its special asset in the shape of its editor, the formidable Carmel
Snow of "The New Look" fame, for her iconic assessment of Christian Dior's
1947 "Corolle" collection which she summed up as "such a new look" (see
Figure 2.10).

In the editorial section of the March issue which starts at page nr. 125,
Carmel Snow is reporting from the Paris Spring Fashion Show (pp. 143–51)
singling out Balenciaga and Dior:

> The midday sweater that Balenciaga presented and tested last year, and
> that all Paris is juggling, has grown into a great new hit, the overblouse.
> At Dior this whole relaxed waistline is climaxed in his delicious pastel
> pleated crepe de chines with their pleated cardigans that reach the hip,
> hug the hip. Here is a whole new conception of outline ... As we watched
> the collections, and I realized we were seeing the waistline drop, I longed
> to say to American women, though you may not like the sound of it, the
> sight of it is wonderful. (1952: 143)

Carmel Snow also alerts us to "the new name to know"—Hubert de
Givenchy:

> Paris has a new young man—Hubert de Givenchy. His boutique clothes
> have won the world. They are modern (many separates) fresh and
> sagacious. He knows to the last *souffle* exactly how far to go. Everyone
> is crazy about his white shirtings—his up cut beach pants—huge chic
> bags—his new approach to colour—his *blanchisserie* ["whites" as the
> English would say]. (1952: 152)

Apart from fashion, the March issue dedicated space to cultural and art issues expertly covered by established writers and artists: the painter Peter Blake on José Luis Sert, here introduced as "one of the world's leading modern architects, president of CIAM (Congrés Internationaux d'Architecture Moderne), and one of the greatest living city planners" (p. 161). Even more impressive is an article written by Arthur Knight on art films (pp. 181–3; pp. 223–4; p. 228) in which the author makes the point that "art films" only emerged in the last ten years but also that this new category was specifically about art, and he singled out the work of a Belgian art critic Paul Haesaerts, who in comparison with his predecessors Luciano Emmer and Enrico Gras

- who working on a shoe string budget produced a long series of stimulating stints on the paintings of such artists as Bosch, Botticelli, Carpaccio, Giotto and Fra Angelico—could develop the genre. Thus his feature length film on Rubens and his shorter film on Picasso, benefited "not only the story of the pictures but, through the pictures the personality of the artist behind them."

This is followed by an accomplished analysis of Haesarts latest film:

In his latest film "From Renoir to Picasso," Haesarts uses all the tricks of the movie medium—split screen, stop motion, animated diagrams, zooming cameras—to contrast and compare three separate tendencies in French art since the turn of the century. Here is ART CRITICISM on a new plane, with pertinent references made immediate and visual, the need for words reduced to a minimum. (Knight, 1952: 223–4)

The twenty-first century: October 2015

Our conclusion can almost be summed in the meek: "How times have changed," and perhaps Karl Marx provides at least one of the explanations in his concept of the "fetishism of the commodities" taken to a perilous extreme by the market economy whose consequence is the operative word: branding! Everything is a brand whose sole value consists of its monetary and not artistic, aesthetic, or even utilitarian value. Many of the "features" in the contemporary fashion press are advertorials, marked in the UK and Australia by a discreet notice "advertising feature," and even the social pages are connected to what marketing calls "contra" or cross-marketing of companies, events, and also people. Instagram, a very interesting tool of communication (developed in 2010 as a free mobile app for photosharing and from 2013 for video), can be used as a very creative and poetic tool, or it can be flooded with ads for those who wish to gain more followers, buy body-building supplements, or book restaurants they have never heard of. It is also used in interesting ways to diarise the daily musings of people

that range from the manufacture of crocodile handbags (@iamethankoh—
Ethan Koh and his family produce crocodile handbags from Singapore) to
young men in Thailand who shop at Dior and Prada (@adisaik—Kuhn Adisai
Kunjara Na Ayudhya—a regular socialite and fashion consumer in *Thai
Tatler*). Today's neo-liberal economy prefers terms such as "strategic plans,"
"integrated approaches," "metrics," and "Key Performance Indicators."
Targets that are not met are now "rephrased" (we learned this term from
the fashion brand H&M's annual report 2016). It is a well-oiled machine in
which the language of contemporary management subsumes "divergence"
and calls retrenchment "back filling" in a callous way unprecedented in
human history.

5

Fashion Journalism: Theory

What is theory?

Theory is the structure which provides the support to a body of academic knowledge so that it can stand up to scrutiny in a manner analogous to the way an architectural structure enables a building to stabilize. In the case of the latter, however, structures are traditionally hidden from view, although we are still wondering how two such pioneering architects as Richard Rogers and Renzo Piano have changed all that with what was to become one of the most iconic building in the world: the museum of modern art, Centre Georges Pompidou, Paris, inaugurated in 1977. What they did was to turn it literally inside out by exposing its infrastructure to the world. The analogy of theory and architecture here holds true, as the circle who developed what we now call "French Theory" were actively engaged in the planning and conceptualization of the "Beaubourg moment" that eventually led to the building of that Parisian cultural center. Yet when we discuss the theoretical basis of most specialized areas of research, which are hidden and need exposing, they appear suspect, or worse still, have their usefulness questioned.

We will start with the ubiquitous question: "What is theory?"—and in order to find the answer, we turn to philosophy, specifically to Aristotle's philosophy. In his *Metaphysics* he distinguishes three kinds of "thought," which put plainly are practical, theoretical, and productive (creative), and he argues that "if all thought is either practical, productive (creative) or theoretical, physics must be a theoretical science" (Aristotle, Metaphysics VI, (E) I, in: Aristotle, 2001: 778). These three forms of "thought" proposed in his classificatory system are knowing (*theoria*), doing (*praxis*), and making (*poiesis*) (Beardsley, 1966: 55), and it is the "knowing" aspect of thought which constitutes the basis of what we refer to as theory or theoretical knowledge.

The British philosopher Gilbert Ryle (1900–1976) famously explained the distinction between theoretical and practical (he left out the Aristotelian "productive," e.g., creative) knowledge by using the expressions "knowing that" and "knowing how" for theoretical and practical knowledge respectively, by starting with the former:

> When we speak of the intellect or, better, of the intellectual powers and performances of persons, we are referring primarily to that special class of operations which constitute theorizing. The goal of these operations is knowledge of true propositions or facts. Mathematics and the established natural sciences are the model accomplishments of human intellects. (Ryle, 1968: 27)

With regard to the second, Ryle makes the point that practical knowledge, e.g., "knowing how" does require intellectual input, but he emphasized that the exercise of intelligence and the practical operation are not discreet entities and cannot—as he put it—be analyzed into "a tandem operation"; rather, we have to argue that "to perform intelligently is to do one thing and not two things" (Ryle, 1968: 41). Ryle gives the example of a boy learning to play chess:

> It should be noticed that the boy is not said to know how to play, if all he can do is to recite the rules accurately. He must be able to make the required moves. But he is said to know how to play, if, although he cannot cite the rules, he normally does make the permitted moves, avoid the forbidden moves and protest if his opponent makes forbidden moves. His knowledge *how* is exercised primarily in the moves that he makes, or concedes, and in the moves that he avoids or vetoes. (Ryle, 1968: 41)

By presenting a "compare/contrast" exercise between "knowing that" and "knowing how" Ryle sums up also the similarities and differences between them:

> There are certain parallelisms between knowing *how* and knowing *that*, as well as certain divergences. We speak of learning how to play an instrument as well as of learning that something is the case; of finding out how to prune trees as well as finding out that the Romans had a camp in a certain place; of forgetting how to tie a reef-knot as well as of forgetting that the German for "knife" is "*Messer*." We can wonder *how* as well as wonder *whether.* (Ryle, 1968: 29)

In 1912, the British philosopher Bertrand Russell (1872–1970) published a slender book entitled *The Problems of Philosophy* that proved an invaluable help in introducing to students the central problems of philosophy. Among them *epistemology* (theory of knowledge) was given pride of place, confirming its centrality in the understanding of the foundations of human civilization and—as such Russell explained in the preface of the book—its importance cannot be overestimated:

In the following pages I have confined myself in the main to those problems of philosophy in regard to which I thought it possible to say something positive and constructive, since merely negative criticism seemed out of place. For this reason, theory of knowledge occupies a larger space than metaphysics in the present volume, and some topics much discussed by philosophers are treated very briefly, if at all. (Russell, 1976: Preface)

Russell's position regarding the centrality of epistemology is confirmed by the list of contents which outlines all the epistemological issues he deals with: "Knowledge by Acquaintance and Knowledge by Description," "On Our Knowledge of general Principles," "How *A Priori* Knowledge is Possible," "On Our Knowledge of Universals," and the last chapter (nr. 13) "Knowledge, Error, and Probable Opinion." In this little book with his characteristic wry humor and wit, Russell introduces the strangeness of philosophical inquiry to the eager beginner, who is left (as we were when we read it) wanting more.

"Theory," however, managed to become a word which instils insecurity in students, and fashion theory is no exception given that the combination between **fashion**, still regarded by many as an industry that is potentially lucrative and ruthless in equal measure and therefore not worth studying at academic level, and the arcane "mysteries" implied by **theory** does not exactly instil confidence in those willing to undertake research.

Fortunately, we have an incipient bibliography for fashion theory whose brave authors/editors took it upon themselves to render the subject approachable and even likeable to students. Two books were published during the same year, 2007 (at that time the only ones in the theory field although sociological studies had also been published), confirming that although "fashion theory" is still a newcomer to the academic field of fashion studies and while its importance cannot be overemphasized, it can also be an enjoyable subject to study. They are Malcolm Barnard (ed.): *Fashion Theory: A Reader,* Routledge, 2007 and Linda Welters and Abby Lillethun: *The Fashion Reader*, Berg, 2007. We have also included the quarterly magazine *Fashion Theory* (*The Journal of Dress, Body and Culture*) started in 1997 by Dr. Valerie Steele—distinguished author and curator of cutting-edge exhibitions and Director of the Museum at FIT (New York).

Initially—as she once told Miller—she intended to provide a forum for academics and researchers to publish academic articles or further develop ideas for books, and this is still the case to date, and although other academic fashion magazines followed suit, *Fashion Theory* still sets the benchmark for academic achievement of this type. When the title appeared it was almost a provocation as no academic journal before it had made such a volley and in its graphic design, interesting cover images (often drawn from private collections, many with a strong feminist angle) and startling contents it was exciting to all those eager to find ways of theorizing the topic of fashion. It is interesting to note how the topic of fashion and its status in the academic world of related subjects, such as the history of art, have changed.

The circle of "costume" historians and theorists of fashion were able to build on achievements laid by many others, including the dress-focused sociological research of Margaret P. Grindereng, Joanne Eicher and their many graduates at the University of Minnesota (Johnson, Torntore, and Eicher), the textile-focused research of those connected with economic history and a charitable organization The Pasold Trust (from 1964), the art historical approach pioneered at the Courtauld Institute by Stella Mary Newton and further developed by Aileen Ribeiro and others, and the expertise of conservation and interlinked museological studies which had grown apace after World War II—the Abegg Stiftung (foundation) in Riggisberg near Bern is the outstanding example.

But it should not come as no surprise that the word "fashion" continues to attract incredulity in many academic circles (and the so-called "fashion academics" who proclaim the debate is concluded are clearly wrong if they go to any large assembly of historians, English Literature, or much of Art History), given that people still regard it as a frivolous pursuit amounting to no more than acquiring the latest "must have" fashion item at an exorbitant price. Many academics, like members of the general public, seem to think that something so commercial cannot be analyzed in any programmatic way (the existence in recent times of two substantial EU-funded research projects, one on transmission of fashion in the early modern era, and one on the "business" of fashion, would seem to show the obverse, but these projects are far from typical).[1] But things are beginning to change and pride of place for her efforts to alter this negative perception of fashion within broader cultural investigation must go to the late Ingrid Sischy (1952–2015), who as editor of the influential *Artforum* dared to place on the cover of the February 1982 issue an outfit by the Japanese fashion designer Issey Miyake, justifying her unprecedented decision by arguing that it was about time the art world welcomed fashion as an integral part of visual culture. Thirty-four years later the *Courtauld Institute of Art* celebrates Dr. Valerie Steele for her contribution to the academic study of fashion. In her acceptance speech she explained how when she expressed an interest to study fashion for her Ph.D. at Yale University, she too was met with incredulity, but instead of being discouraged she became even more determined to pursue an academic career in the subject.

---

[1]*Fashioning the Early Modern*, 2010–2013; see http://www.fashioningtheearlymodern.ac.uk. *The Enterprise of Culture: International Structures and Connections in the Fashion Industry Since 1945*, 2013–2016; see http://www.enterpriseofculture.leeds.ac.uk.

Fashion theory: Do we need it?

The anthology edited by Malcolm Barnard (ed.), *Fashion Theory: A Reader* provides a valuable collection of texts by past and present authors whose writings were deemed to qualify as theoretical tools for the fashion researcher, starting with Karl Marx and Sigmund Freud. Both of them provided two seminal methodologies (tools) of research for the fashion theorist that were related to the concept of "fetishism"; the former predicated of commodities and the latter analyzed as a pathological symptom defined by Freud as a fear of castration. By studying these two texts students not only gain unexpected insights into the hidden mechanisms that control fashion but they enable them to understand how to choose and apply a theoretical framework to their own case studies. As it happens, students are familiar with how commodities are fetishized at the expense of their bank accounts when a Prada bag is priced at thousands of pounds. They might not know that the mechanisms which contribute to this situation can be explained through what Marx calls the "quasi-mystical" character of the "product of labour as soon as it assumes the form of a commodity," which you might understand as "branding," but Marx calls it "fetishism": "I call this the fetishism which attaches itself to the products of labour as soon as they are produced as commodities, and is therefore inseparable from the production of commodities" (Marx, in Barnard, 2007: 348). "Fetishism" and fashion return in the context of eroticism and Barnard lists Sigmund Freud's "Fetishism"; David Kunzle's "The Special Historic and Psychological Role of Tight-Lacing" (MS dated 1977 and subsequent writings); and Valerie Steele's *Fetish: Fashion, Sex and Power* (Oxford University Press 1996), a subject to which she made a significant contribution over the years.

Linda Welters and Abby Lillethun also provide an anthology, but as its title indicates, their remit is wider, including topics as "Brief History of Modern fashion" (starting with the Enlightenment), "Fashion and Identity," "The Geography of Dress," "Politics of Fashion," "Fashion and the Body," "Fashion and Art," "Fashion in the Media," "From Haute couture to the Street," "The Fashion Business," and finally the "Future of Fashion." Their imaginative and wide-ranging subject areas indicate the multiple ways in which fashion can be encountered and studied.

Only one of its eleven parts—Part II—is dedicated to "Fashion Theory" (pp. 77–120), consisting of an introduction contributed by Abby Lillethun, followed by six chapters—Kurt Lang and Gladys Engel Lang: "The Power of Fashion," Roland Barthes: "Written Clothing," Grant McCracken: "The Fashion System," "Joanne Entwistle": "The Dressed Body," Sandra Niessen: "Re-Orienting Fashion Theory" and Caroline Evans: "Fashion at the Edge," some of which are extracts from books, as in the case of Roland Barthes's chapter taken from his book, "The Fashion System" first published in 1967.

Definition and explanation of the terms involved: Fashion, theory, fashion theory

A useful approach to understanding how fashion and theory got together so to speak to become "Fashion Theory" is to look at them individually:

Fashion

Perhaps, we can start by paraphrasing Gertrude Stein's celebrated aphorism: "A rose, is a rose, is a rose" and say: "fashion is fashion is fashion," simply meaning that things are such as they are, and we have Welters and Lillethun quoting all of the key costume historians: François Boucher, James Laver, Christopher Breward, and Tortora and Eubank, not so much to provide a definition of fashion but to establish its inception. When was fashion born? To their list of researchers we can add a later contribution: an essay by Sarah Grace Heller entitled "The Birth of Fashion" (Heller in Riello and McNeil, 2010: 25–39), which is a useful summing up of the various answers provided by scholars to this question. While she does not hope to solve the question by providing an identifiable starting point, a rather more pragmatic conclusion is reached whereby it is not possible to assign a "birth date" to fashion; instead, we need to accept a multiplicity of "births":

> The conclusion to which we must return is that fashion seems to stage its own birth again and again, because a fundamental characteristic of fashion is declaring the past invalid in favour of a new, improved present. Fashion is a phoenix, constantly dying and reincarnating itself. (Heller in Riello and McNeil, 2010: 34)

While it is not possible to identify a "birth" date for fashion, what enables each and every stage of its "reincarnation" is that a "fashion system" is already in position, and one example is Burgundian fashion made possible by such a "fashion system" which enabled the changes in male fashion at the Burgundian court during the fourteenth century:

> Fashion would stage many more would-be births in the centuries that followed, always gaining momentum with new technologies and greater populations affected. The radical change in male dress that was staged by the young men of the wealthy fourteenth century Burgundian court could only have happened because a fashion system was already in place, just as with the adoption of the new poetry. From *pourpoint* to poetic form, fashionable objects change, always multiplying, always seeming newly invented; but the desire to consume them and invent them has been steadily present in the West for at least eight centuries. (Heller in Riello and McNeil, 2010: 34–50)

Malcolm Barnard chose a different route to explain fashion, and with typical attention to structural clarity, divided the introduction into four sections starting with his aims and objectives: "What is this book about?" to which the answer provided is: "It is about the theories (or organised ideas) behind what we think, write and say about the things we wear" (Barnard, 2007: 1).

In the second section dedicated to "Fashion," instead of an historical overview Barnard provides an approach which borrows from such diverse disciplines as cultural studies, sociology, and anthropology, but ultimately Barnard settled for Anne Hollander's minimalist definition:

[E]verybody has to get dressed in the morning and go about the day's business ... what everybody wears to do this has taken different forms in the West for about seven hundred years and that is what fashion is. (Hollander in Barnard, 2007: 3)

It is important to note that Hollander was writing her innovative arguments much earlier than is often recognized, partly due to the influence of her magisterial *Seeing through Clothes* (1978). Her literary approach in that influential work dates from articles written in the early 1970s.

Theory

While Welters and Lillethun do not much address the concept of theory, Barnard certainly does, in the third section of his Introduction by starting with Aristotle, who was the first to define the concept. But what is worth mentioning is a lovely example that Barnard gives: "the well known story concerning the farmer, the general and the art student standing together in a field":

Asked to describe what they see, each gives an entirely different account. The farmer sees a profitable unit with good drainage, which would be easy to plough and would support arable crops. The general sees an exposed killing field that would be impossible to defend. And the art student sees a pastoral scene that would make a delightful watercolour if the trees on the left were a darker shade of green and moved a little to the right. (Barnard, 2007: 5)

What does this story tell us? It explains in a charming way what we knew all along: namely that different methodologies (tools) can be applied to the same object of analysis. We have a given object (a field) assessed from three different vantage points: that of the farmer, of the general, and of the art student:

Looking at the field, each sees something different, according to the conceptual frameworks they adopt: to this extent, what they see is a product of the theories they are accustomed to using. The farmer is employing a combination of economics, biology and geology to produce what one might call agricultural theory; the general is employing military theory, and the student is employing aesthetic theory. (Barnard, 2007)

Barnard further references an important epistemological issue, regarding "facts" that he appears to be using interchangeably with "truths" which constitute the two equivalent terms of what philosophers call "the correspondence theory of truth," which goes according to philosopher A. D. Woozley something like this:

> I propose hereafter, in discussing the Correspondence theory, to speak of a proposition as being one term of the relation, as being that which is wanted to correspond with whatever make the belief in question true. (Woozley, 1967: 131)

Barnard refers to "the theory-ladenness" of "facts" or the "theory-dependency of what is ostensibly innocent observation," whereby:

> To the farmer, it is true, or a fact, that the field will support arable crops; to the general, it is a true fact that the field is impossible to defend; and to the art student it is a fact that they imagined watercolour would be improved by moving the trees.

Consequently, Barnard argued, "each of the facts however is a product of the theory that is being used, or dependent upon it" (Barnard, 2007: 5).

What is actually happening is that "facts" themselves, as the second term of the correspondence equation that makes a proposition true or false, are a debatable concept. "The field yields arable crops" is true if the arability of the field is a "fact." But what is a fact? Woozley introduced a new term—"event"—defined as a spatio-temporal occurrence, giving as an example "the dropping of the atom bomb on Hiroshima in August 1945," but we also note that it is a fact (true) that an atomic bomb was dropped on Hiroshima on such a such a date and time; thus, "the fact is a conveniently intelligible aspect of the event, the way an event looks to a mind thinking about it" (Woozley, 1967: 132), and it is therefore clear that facts and not events are the second term in a correspondence theory. Barnard is right to argue that "facts" are not out there in the world but in our minds, or as Woozley put it, facts are the way our mind thinks about events.

Fashion theory

Unlike Malcolm Barnard, who considers the terms "fashion" and "theory" separately, and then turns to "fashion theory," Welters and Lillethun focus on fashion theory by starting with the perennial question:

What is fashion theory? A theory consists of a conceptual network of propositions that explain an observable phenomenon. While fashion is an "observable phenomenon" at this time no comprehensive theory of fashion has been universally accepted. Instead, concepts and propositions concerning fashion have been suggested from a variety of disciplinary perspectives. (Welters and Lillethun, 2007: 77)

An important point is made here, namely that because the very nature of fashion is change—this is why "a unifying fashion theory has not developed because the very place that fashion exists—within culture—transforms swiftly and continuously" (Welters and Lillethun, 2007: 77).

The authors mention some of the "classical" theorists such as Thorstein Veblen who criticized the "leisure classes for their conspicuous consumption," and of course we are aware that his comments influenced by Marxism can only be applicable to the social and economic conditions of nineteenth-century society. He was followed by Georg Simmel, whose "trickle down" theory postulated that in a stratified capitalist society, the wealthy provided the model for the poor classes who emulated them. Simmel was followed by G. A. Field, who reversed the process in what came to be known as "trickle up theory," called by social-anthropologist Ted Polhemus' "bubble up": same thing/different disciplines. Polhemus is a good example of a theorist who was in the "field" (his field was the street and club culture of the 1970s and 1980s) and was able to make his ideas accessible to very large audiences through his invaluable photography and pithy descriptions (he is now also a novelist having published *BOOM!* and a blogger: see http://www. tedpolhemus.com/index.html)[2] (Figure 5.1). Many important texts written by feminists, including Elizabeth Wilson (*Adorned in Dreams*, 1985) and Minna Thornton and Caroline Evans (*Women and Fashion: A New Look*, 1989), were similarly produced in the "field" of observing contemporary women (including themselves) interact with personal wardrobes, explore museum exhibits, and stroll in the street and the club. Finally, we come to the recent development of "a prominent research paradigm," namely structuralism, and while the above historical examples of theoretical approaches are not included in this volume, structuralist theory is—with Roland Barthes.

A special mention in Welters and Lillethun's section dedicated to theory is fashion which has been extensively dealt with in a number of contexts, starting with what is probably the best known but least understood example: Roland Barthes's notoriously difficult *The Fashion System*, first published in 1967. In it Barthes proposes a system of meaning within which fashion must be analyzed, namely structuralism, and then proceeds to show how

---

[2]BOOM! See http://www.tedpolhemus.com/boom.html.

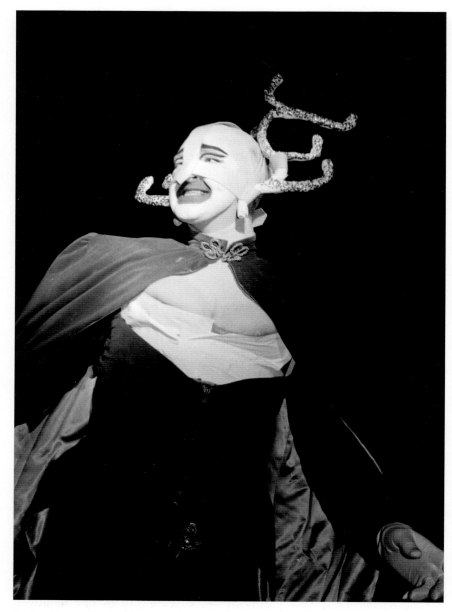

FIGURE 5.1 *Ted Polhemus, photographer, Leigh Bowery presenting fashion show in the Slaughter House Gallery, Smithfield Market, London, 1987, with designs by Dean Bright, Rachel Auburn, and Andre Walker. © Ted Polhemus.*

clothes are analyzed, specifically fashion magazines both as visual images and written text, e.g., a dress becomes a photograph and a dress becomes a written text; two different systems referencing the same object. This is famously summed in the paragraph with which Barthes opened chapter I, entitled "Written Clothing," as discussed by us in Chapter 4. Fortunately, for the students of fashion theory, Barthes has been analyzed elsewhere in depth, one example being Michael Carter, from whom we also find out that "Barthes" reputation as a "fashion thinker" rests mainly upon the doctorate that never was, *The Fashion System*, which explains its inaccessibility: "It has to be said that the book is one of the less seductive examples of Barthes's writing and has been variously described as 'rebarbative' ('unattractive and objectionable') and 'structuralism's *Moby Dick*'" (Carter, 2006: 144). The exception to the 300 or so pages of this heavy tome is the *Introduction*, in which Barthes explains his methodology employed in answering the question "What is fashion?," but as Carter points out, the crucial word in this context is "system," defined as "a group or set of related or associated material or immaterial things forming a unity or complex whole" which lay at the heart of the revolution that swept through French intellectual life after the Second World War and one which has come to be known by the generic term "structuralism", "system", "structure" and "totality" which are all closely related terms (Carter, 2006: 144). In this sweep we arrive back at the Plateau Beaubourg in Paris and its Centre Pompidou (conceived c. 1970, built 1977), and its radical attempt inspired by philosophers, including Gilles Deleuze to rethink the foundation of both museum user-experience (the visitor) and objecthood (the way in which things are exhibited there in a "kinetic" manner) (Holden, 2008; Wilson, 2010).

If a system is, according to Roland Barthes, defined as: "a group or set of related or associated material or immaterial things forming a unity or complex whole" (Carter, 2006: 144) why can we not, instead of "system" use the old-fashioned term "culture"?, itself a maddeningly complicated term. We turn to the esteemed *A Dictionary of Cultural and Critical Theory* where we find a useful working definition of culture as: "A term of virtually limitless application, which initially may be understood to refer to everything that is produced by human beings as distinct from all that is part of nature" (Payne, 1997: 128). What is interesting here is that among the wealth of scholars and writers listed as having dealt with the concept of culture, including Claude Lévi-Strauss, Raymond Williams, Homi Bhabha, Pierre Bourdieu, and many others, Clifford Geertz's definition comes closest to our suggestion that what Barthes called a "system," and the notion of "culture" amount to a very similar (sameness is too dangerous to use here) thing because it was Clifford Geertz who defines culture by way of semiotics as "the web of significance" spun by human beings' (Geertz in Payne, 1997: 128). That Carter was trained as an anthropologist should be highlighted here, as it colored his different perspectives on fashion/dress/

costume, and his important publications, some of which were printed by small presses that can be difficult to obtain (Carter 2013—*Overdressed: Barthes, Darwin & the Clothes that Speak*, Puncher & Wattman, Sydney).

Grant McCracken tried to throw light on how we might interpret the fashion system, which he defined as one of the instruments for "meaning movement" comparable to advertising, which he wrote is "less frequently observed, studied, and understood as an instrument of meaning" (McCracken in Welters and Lillethun, 2007: 90). He identifies three "distinct ways" in which the fashion world (he appears to use "world" interchangeably with system) transfers meaning to goods. In its first capacity, "the fashion system performs a transfer of meaning from the culturally constituted world to consumer goods that is remarkably similar in character and effect to the transfer performed by advertising." In its second capacity, "the fashion system actually invents new cultural meanings in a modest way. This invention is undertaken by 'opinion leaders' who help shape and refine existing cultural meaning, encouraging the reform of cultural categories and principles."

In its third capacity "the fashion system engages not just in the invention of cultural meanings but also in its radical reform" (McCracken in Welters and Lillethun, 2007: 90–1).

The conclusion reached by McCracken is nice and simple:

In short, both advertising and the fashion system are instruments for transfer of meaning from the culturally and historically constituted world to consumer goods. They are two of the means by which meaning is invested in the "object code." It is thanks to them that the objects of our world carry such a richness, variety, and versatility of meaning and can serve us so variously in acts of self-definition and social communication (McCracken in Welters and Lillethun, 2007: 92).

We turn now to Barnard, who asks this very question "What is fashion theory?" in the last section of the Introduction, and he too concurs as to its polysemic nature:

There is no one set of ideas or a single conceptual framework with which fashion might be defined, analysed and critically explained. Consequently, there is no single discipline, approach or discrete body of work that can be identified and presented here as fashion theory. Rather, there are theories about fashion, or, to put it another way, there are fashion theories. (Barnard, 2007: 7)

Like Welters and Lillethun, Barnard, too, proceeds to single out "which disciplines and which theories might be applied to fashion" (Barnard, 2007: 7) and to that effect selected a few examples he considered seminal, starting with Fernand Braudel, Lisa Tickner, Elizabeth Wilson, Gilles Lipovetsky, and finally Lou Taylor and Valerie Steele, both of whom are supporters of "the idea of an 'object-based history'" (2007: 7). The conclusion offered by Barnard is that the selection of theories useful to fashion comes from the same source: the humanities and social sciences, as his selection of tests is concerned:

> with explaining and understanding (the meanings) of fashion: it is therefore a humanities/social science reader. The essays that are collected here are from the disciplines that make up the humanities and social sciences because they all deal, in their own ways, with the explanation and understanding of the objects, institutions, personnel and practices of fashion. (Barnard, 2007: 9)

How to apply theory to practice: Case study

We selected an example that demonstrates how a theoretical framework finds application in a fashion context by using a book which excels in this practice, Caroline Evans's *Fashion at the Edge*, published by Yale University Press in 2003. Its subtitle "Spectacle, Modernity and Deathliness" outlines the three main areas of research on which the book is focused, and among them the first is of particular relevance, because in the 1990s, which is the historical period analyzed through these headings, "spectacle" achieved special prominence. There was a remarkable shift which changed the discreet system of presenting collections to esteemed clients behind closed doors. Christian Dior's historic "Corolle" line, famously nick-named "The New Look" by the indomitable fashion editor of *Harper's Bazaar* Carmel Snow on February 12, 1947, when it was shown at Maison Christian Dior, Paris, is a prime example. But all this was to change, and radical change was brought about largely by three fashion designers, building on the transition to a new fashion paradigm created also by the role of the Japanese in Paris in the 1980s: John Galliano, Alexander McQueen, and Hussein Chalayan in the 1990s.

To that effect the fashion show mutated into a *spectacle* which could be approximated with equivalents from the art world, such as performance art, and it must be agreed that what Galliano or McQueen presented was in no way inferior or less "spectacular" than Yves Klein's (1928–1963) "Leap into Void," literally choreographed in 1960 when the maverick artist (who also happened to be a judo black belt) was photographed by the Hungarian photographer János Kender in the process of jumping from the second floor of a private house in the Paris suburb of *Fontenay aux Roses*. Evans brings into focus the Marxist Guy Debord's (1931–1994) book *The Society of Spectacle* given that, Evans argues:

> In French *spectacle* also means theatrical presentation and the fashion show is undoubtedly a part of Debord's "society of spectacle" in the way that it transforms commercial enterprise into dazzling, display, aestheticising everyday life on the catwalks. (Evans, 2003: 73)

In the section "Modelling Alienation" (pp. 177–83), Alexander McQueen's Spring/Summer 1999 chosen for analysis is described as follows:

> The show was opened by the athlete and model Aimee Mullins in a pair of hand-carved prosthetic legs designed by McQueen (the model was born without shin bones and had her legs amputated below the knee at the age of one), and closed by the model Shalom Harlow who revolved like a music-doll on a turntable as her white dress was sprayed acid green and black by two menacing industrial paint sprayers which suddenly came to life on the catwalk. (Evans, 2003: 177)

This is "what the eyes see" at a fashion show, but the fashion journalist cannot just provide a description, however scintillating it appears to the eyes. That also would be less than adequate at professional level. It falls to the fashion journalist to provide an analysis, even a critical analysis of what is going on and in order to do so a theoretical framework (vantage point) appropriate for the example needs to be selected. This is of course the most challenging aspect, because it falls to the reporter/writer to match the right theory to the event that needs to be written about, and Evans provides an excellent example of how this is done by moving on from the descriptive to the analytical:

> Juxtaposing the organic with the inorganic (a model that mimicked a doll, a paint sprayer that mimicked human motions and an artificial leg that enhanced human performance) the collection skewed the relation of object and subject to evoke Marx's commodity exchange in which "people and things trade semblances: social relations take on the character" of object relations and commodities assume the active agency of people. In the figures of these two young women the ghosts of Marx and Lukács seemed to flutter up and live again at the end of the twentieth century, as the embodied forms of alienation, reification and commodity fetishism. (Evans, 2003: 177)

Evans does not say, and this is the crucial point, that alienation, reification, and commodity fetishism are either the rightful or only theoretical frameworks that can get to the bottom of McQueen's fashion show; rather, she writes: "the collection skewed the relation of object and subject to evoke Marx's commodity exchange." Here we need to emphasize the words "to evoke" as the key which opens the door to our understanding of how a case-study (example) is matched to possible frameworks which can work well but are by no means the only ones that can be selected.

Once the theoretical frameworks *alienation*, *reification*, and *commodity fetishism* are selected for explaining purposes we can proceed by taking a close look at her choice and see if we are happy with it, and if so, how is our understanding of McQueen's show enhanced.

Reification

The concept of "reification" comes from Latin: *res* means thing and *facere* is to make, hence "to make a thing." In Marxist studies, it is an alternative to "alienation" whereby the worker is reduced to the status of a mechanical tool, touchingly exemplified in Charlie Chaplin's film 1936 film *Modern Times*, in which the lovable but hapless character of Chaplin's "tramp" works on the assembly line and ends by having a nervous breakdown.

The breakdown between the division man/machine was also captured on the poster where we see a full length frontal image of a frozen Chaplin holding the machinery he is meant to use in his hands raised at shoulder level so as to frame his head: a brutal blending of man-machine almost were it not for Chaplin's frightened and very human eyes.

Alienation

The concept of "alienation" itself is at the basis of Marx's philosophy as it turns up in *The Philosophical Manuscripts of 1844* in which Marx argues that the more wealth the worker produces in the capitalist society, the poorer he becomes, in fact he becomes "an ever cheaper commodity the more commodities he creates":

> This fact expresses merely that the object which labour produces—labour product—confronts it as *something alien*, as a *power independent* of the producer. The product of labour is labour which has been congealed in an object, which has become material: it is the *objectification* of labour. Labour's realization is its objectification. In the conditions dealt with by political economy this realization of labour appears as *loss of reality* for the workers, objectification as *loss of the object* and *object-bondage*; appropriation as *estrangement* as *alienation*. (Marx in Appleby et al., 1996: 169)

The dire consequences are that in this process the worker loses touch with reality "to the point," Marx argued with a peculiar sense of black humor, to that of "starving to death." We see another dire consequence with Charlie Chaplin, for whom the assembly line became a treat to his sanity, resulting in a nervous break-down and so, Marx concluded: "All these consequences are contained in the definition that the worker is related to the *product of his labour* as to an *alien* object" (Appleby et al., 1996).

The fetishism of the commodities

This process of separation between man and the product of his labor which constitutes the basis of alienation finds application in Marx's distinction between the "use" and "exchange" value of an object thus transformed into a commodity, summed up the brilliant Marxist philosopher Terry Eagleton:

It is in the concept of use-value, above all, that Marx deconstructs the opposition between the practical and the aesthetic. When he writes of the emancipated senses as "theoreticians in their immediate praxis," he means that *theoria*, the pleasurable contemplation of an object's material qualities, is an active process within our functional relations with it. We experience the sensuous wealth of things by drawing them within our signifying projects—a stance which differs on the one hand from the crude instrumentalism of exchange-value, and on the other hand from some disinterested aesthetic speculation. (Eagleton, 1992: 205)

An analysis of capitalist economy was developed by Marx in *Capital*, volume I (first published in German in 1867), where he analyzed the interrelated concepts of "commodities" and "exchange." Marx traced back processes of exchange to the simplest form such as "use" value: "the desire to enjoy the peculiar properties of a particular good":

The simplest form of exchange is barter: you have something I want, I have something you want. We agree to swap. What we each seek is the use-value embodied in the objects of exchange. The aim of the economic relationship is to enjoy the sensuous use of the object sought. Even if money is brought into equation as the means by which exchange is effected it does not affect the start and end point of the process which, in each case is use-value. (Hampsher-Monk, 1992: 540)

But in capitalist society all this changes with the replacement of "use value" with that of "exchange value":

Capitalism begins and ends with exchange value—money, credit, a bank balance, which is not inherently consumable. The purpose of capitalist relations is to increase exchange value, not to enjoy use. It is a kind of fetishist, compulsive behaviour on a social scale. (Hampsher-Monk, 1992)

Chapter 29 in Barnard's book dedicated to Karl Marx (pp. 347–350) is entitled "The Fetishism of the Commodity and Its Secret"; we are not given the exact source of the extract but it comes from *Capital* and we will provide the full bibliographical reference:

Capital, Part I: "Commodities and Money," chapter 1: Commodities, Section 4: "The Fetishism of the Commodities and the Secret Thereof," pp. 47–59, first translated into English in 1887, pdf. (first published by Progress Publishers, Moscow, USSR, latest proofing: Dave Allinson, 2015)

The fragment selected by Barnard starts with Marx's explanation of the "use value" of an object, exemplified by the artisan creation of a wooden table, "an ordinary sensuous thing" which is altered as soon as the table emerges as "commodity" which in turn confers upon it a "mystical character."

Whence, then arises the enigmatic character of the product of labour, as soon as it assumes the form of a commodity? Clearly, it arises from this form (the social form) itself ... The mysterious character of the commodity-form consists therefore simply in the fact that the commodity reflects the social characteristics of men's own labour as objective characteristics of the products of labour themselves, as the socio-natural properties of these things. (Marx in Barnard, 2007: 348)

At this level, the enjoyable sensuousness attached to the "use value" become also "supra-sensible" or "social" values and as with "the misty realm of religion," Marx argued whereby 'the products of the human brain appear as autonomous figures endowed with a life of their own', the same happens to commodities which too acquire an autonomous existence:

So it is with the world of commodities with the products of men's hands I call this the fetishism which attaches itself to the products of labour as soon as they are produced as commodities, and is therefore inseparable from the production of commodities. (Barnard, 2007: 348)

Conclusion

To what extent has Caroline Evans's choice of matching Alexander McQueen's Spring/Summer 1999 show with the Marxist terms of reification, alienation, and commodity fetishism thrown additional light on McQueen's decision to start and end the show with two uncharacteristic models: an athlete with prosthetic legs, Aimee Mullins, and a model, Shalom Harlow, mimicking a doll whose white dress was sprayed by machines? Did the subjective nature of the choice make the theoretical frameworks selected less relevant? The answer is that Evans allowed us new insights into McQueen and the whole period of the 1990s. She gained her insights from theory. She also nowhere suggests that she alone has the right theory or set of theories. Fashion theory, although a new addition to other theories from which it shamelessly borrowed for its own use, only follows an already established practice which can even be applied to the rigorous approach of natural sciences; namely that more than one theory can be applied equally successfully to the same situation or object as Malcolm Barnard's example of the field analyzed from the perspective of the farmer, the military leader, and the art student demonstrates.

6

Fashion Journalism: Practice

Hard news?

In our introduction we have examined the main categories of print journalism. In this second part of the book we will apply them to fashion by starting here with "hard news" and commence our inquiry with a question: can we really talk about hard news in the context of fashion journalism?

Hard news is the most venerable as well as highly specialized category in print journalism. Most importantly, while every category of journalism can be transformed into its corresponding fashion category, if we append fashion to hard news, we have (once again) an oxymoron. We all love a good oxymoron and literature abounds with examples such as *festina lente* (make haste slowly) or the grandest oxymoron of them all: William Shakespeare's immortal, "Love is such sweet sorrow"! This is all very well when the oxymoron is kept where it belongs—a figure of speech—but in this context what we sense is that fashion and news don't make good bedfellows.

To demonstrate our point we turn to Julie Bradford's book *Fashion Journalism*. In it she dedicates two sections to news and feature writing: "Writing news" (pp. 109–13) and "Writing features" (pp. 113–18). We shall start with the former in which she introduces news as a seminal category in journalism, providing an analysis of its well-established structuring rules:

> News stories have a style and structure all of their own, developed over the years to convey information in the quickest, clearest and most attention-grabbing way possible. (Bradford, 2015: 109)

Among the established rules, Bradford references the "news angle," citing the analysis of Lynette Sheridan Burns's book *Understanding Journalism* (2002). What Sheridan Burns argues is that "news writing always starts with the most important *fact*"; thus—she rightly pointed out—when a football match becomes an item of news, the news reporter starts with what is the most important aspect: the score. What she does not mention is that in order for a football match to make it to the front page as news, rather than as reportage/feature, it needs to have something unusual (worthy of news) about it!

Bradford then makes the move from hard to fashion news:

> The same holds true for all types of fashion news stories. If Karl Lagerfeld were to give an interview during which he criticised a public figure's face body or dress sense—as he has been known to do—the news story would begin with the gist of the controversial comment. The second paragraph might give more detail, perhaps with a direct quote … Further down the story, we'd get more quotes, more background on other times the designer has been less than flattering about people … perhaps some angry reaction from fans and a right of reply for balance. (Bradford, 2015: 110–11)

Bradford follows this up by discussing some of the established approaches to news writing, e.g., "the angle" (pp. 110–11), and in the case of Lagerfeld the angle is important because it controls the vantage point from which the news is reported: "The most important or interesting fact at the start is called the *angle*. All stories and reviews are reported from an angle, it highlights what's new or interesting or important about the story, and why we should read it" (Bradford, 2015: 111). She then introduces the "inverted pyramid" structure used in news writing.

The "inverted pyramid" of news simply means that the important details and angles are at the start of the story, narrowing down to minor details and side issues by the end (Bradford, 2015: 112). Finally, "The news intro" (pp. 111–12) is crucial because, Bradford argues, "the intro has to give the most interesting part of the story, the angle, in a nutshell and grab the reader's attention at the same time" (Bradford, 2015: 111).

Before analyzing how, in Bradford's opinion, hard news becomes "fashion news," we will discuss a very thorough account of news writing provided by Wynford Hicks in his book *Writing for Journalists* (pp. 10–44), where he starts with the all important question: "What is news?" The answer is short, sharp, and to the point! "To be news, something must be factual, new and interesting." Above all, "There must be facts to report—without them there can be no news. The facts must be new—to your readers at least. And these facts must be likely to interest your readers" (Hicks et al., 2008: 10).

But his crucial point is that the two "most quoted formulas in the traditional approach to news writing" are firstly Rudyard Kipling's "six questions," which have become the "mantra" in journalism, and secondly, the "news pyramid," which is also known as "the inverted pyramid."

Kipling's questions can be found in one of the stories entitled "The Elephant's Child," published in his charming volume of children's stories entitled "Just so Stories" (1902), which ends with a poem whose opening paragraph is:

> I keep six honest serving-men
> (They taught me all I knew)
> Their names are what and why and when
> and how and where and who.
> (taken from Project Gutenberg EBook of "Just so Stories" (2008, last updated 2013))

Kipling's questions were enthusiastically adopted in journalism and Hicks provides the following textbook example:

> Lady Godiva (WHO) rode (WHAT) naked (HOW) through the streets of Coventry (WHERE) yesterday (WHEN) in a bid to cut taxes (WHY). (Hicks et al., 2008: 13)

These questions, Hicks says, are "facetiously called the clothesline intro—because you can hang everything on it," but they are useful when writing a news story, and in this context "who and what" are particularly relevant:

> Two of these questions—who and what—are obviously essential. In all news intros somebody or something must do or experience something. A useful distinction can be made between "who" stories, in which the focus is on the person concerned, and "what" stories, which are dominated by what happens. (Hicks et al., 2008: 14)

The second is the news (inverted) pyramid and we liked his humorous definition:

> This particular pyramid is not quite as old as the ancient Egyptians. But as a formula for analysing, teaching and practising news writing it goes back a long way ... The purpose of the pyramid is to show that the points in a news story are made in descending order of importance. News is written so that readers can stop reading when they have satisfied their curiosity—without worrying that something important is being held back. To put it another way, news is written so that subeditors can cut stories from the bottom up—again without losing something important. (Hicks et al., 2008)

We return now to fashion journalism to offer a *paragone* (a comparison) between the examples provided by Hicks and by Bradford which will make our point. We will use two examples from Hicks: the first from the *Daily Telegraph* entitled "Man killed as L-driver [leaner-driver] car plunges off cliff," and the sombre opening paragraph says it all:

A man was feared dead last night after his car ran off a 150ft cliff into rough seas when his girlfriend lost control while he was giving her a driving lesson. The woman, in her early 20s scrambled from the Ford Fiesta as it crashed through a low stone wall at the edge of a car park at the Beacon, St. Agnes, on the north Cornwall coast. Andrew Dunklin, 25, from St. Agnes, was trapped in the vehicle as it rolled over the cliff. It is thought he was thrown through the windscreen into the sea.

As Hicks pointed out, "This is a stark and terrible story simply told. The reporter has no need to strain for effect here" (Hicks et al., 2008: 42).

The second example comes from a tabloid the *Daily Mail*. The story may be called dramatic rather than tragic because it deals with human folly. Unlike the first example published in a "broadsheet"—and although they are both "hard news"—it can be argued that even in news journalism there are many degrees of just how "hard" the news can be. The *Daily Mail* example is entitled "Hobbies put judge on the road to ruin" and the story is about John Aspinall QC. This is the opening paragraph:

A judge's entry in Who's Who listed his passions as cars and drinking with friends. Yesterday these twin interests landed John Aspinall QC in court, where he was banned from the road for two and a half years for drink-driving.

This does not sound too bad, but we find out about the serious consequences of this incident several paragraphs further down:

Now his career is in tatters. He has resigned as a crown court recorder, a part-time judge, and faces a Bar Council disciplinary hearing which could mean being suspended from practising as a barrister or even thrown out of the profession. (Hicks et al., 2008: 43)

On this occasion Hicks qualifies this example as "an example of modern news writing, which grabs the reader's attention, then keeps it by answering their questions" (Hicks et al., 2008: 44).

From Bradford we chose also two examples of news, both from tabloids one of which is about Karl Lagerfeld. The first, also from the *Daily Mail*, has the following introduction: "Karl Lagerfeld has provoked fury by labelling pop superstar Adele 'fat'" (Sparks and Todd, 2012 in Bradford, 2015: 111). This is analyzed by Bradford as follows: "It names two protagonists, gets straight to the heart of the row and hints at the reaction, all in 11 words" (Bradford, 2015: 111).

The second is from *The Sun:* "Controversial fashion brand American Apparel has been told to remove a series of images from its website—after a watchdog ruled they were 'overtly sexual'" (Sayer 2013, in Bradford, 2015: 111). In this instance, Bradford argues:

It sums up the most important point of the story—the ban—while adding the "sexual" angle, which is guaranteed to get the reader's attention. It names the brand, with a short description in case its readers aren't familiar with it, but does not name the watchdog until the second paragraph. (Bradford, 2015)

And herein lies the difference: a tragic death in an accident, the self-destruction of a highly accomplished human being who succumbed to wanton pride (hubris) is the stuff that hard news is made of! We found in fact further confirmation in a recent example, the front page of the *Financial Times* (Saturday January 30/Sunday January 31, 2016). We have three main news stories which share the front page and deal with the following factual information reported in a straightforward, matter of fact style:

The first, "Critics hit at slow response to Zika crisis," dealing with the destructive virus spread by mosquitoes summed up to perfection in the opening paragraph:

A specialist fumigates a graveyard in the outskirts of the Peruvian capital Lima to combat Zika, the mosquito-borne virus that has been linked to devastating birth defects and neurological problems in adults.

The second, "Japan joins the negative rates club," which has the subtitle "Move sparks surge in equities and bonds; Fears rise over China and risk of slowdown," was written by three FT correspondents: Robin Harding in Tokyo, Sam Fleming in Washington, and Claire Jones in Frankfurt, which adds to the impeccability of the information contained in the report, summed up in the opening paragraph as follows:

The Bank of Japan has cut interest rates to minus 0.1 per cent, stunning analysts and sparking a surge in equity and bond markets, as policymakers around the world respond to mounting worries about the outlook in China and the risks of a global slowdown;

The third by Tim Bradshaw reporting from San Francisco is entitled "Apple builds secret virtual reality unit in search of the next big tech platform," and it opens as follows:

Apple has assembled a large team of experts in virtual and augmented reality and built prototypes of headsets that could one day rival Facebook's Oculus Rift or Microsoft's Hololens, as it seeks new sources of growth beyond the iPhone.

This is news reporting at its best, but above all it complies with what Wynford Hicks, and in fact every news journalist around the globe knows:

"News must be factual, new and interesting" (Hicks et al., 2008: 10), the operative word here being **factual**.

We turn next to the two examples provided by Julie Bradford. Some might comment that the concept of the *paragone* is unfair, because of such different readerships of the publications under discussion, and this is certainly true from the point of view of the content. While a *Daily Mail* reader might be less interested in the arcane technology of a mega company such as *Apple* or the movement of equity and bond markets, the *Daily Mail* also needs to provide hard news like everybody else, and they do. But the example referencing Karl Lagerfield is something else. The Lagerfeld story has not provided any news based upon facts. Instead, it offered a biased interpretation of a ridiculous situation. Notwithstanding the monumental triviality of the "scandal," we wish to demonstrate that this has nothing to do with hard news, and to prove it, we turn to a structural analysis.

In the *Daily Mail* example that opens with the statement "Karl Lagerfeld has produced fury but labelling pop superstar Adele 'fat' " nothing happens at all! Some people are furious, some are not, some probably laugh at such stupidity but what is important is the way that the word "fat" is interpreted. Had it been used in seventeenth-century Belgium, Adele might have been pleased to be seen as a Rubenesque voluptuous beauty. In the cultural context of the twenty-first century however, this reads as an insult. Why? As Malcolm Barnard explains in the introduction of his book *Fashion Theory: A Reader*, it is about theory:

> It (the book) is about the theories (or organised ideas) behind what we think, write and say about the things we wear: When, for example, we mock our male friends for wearing a shirt that is a bit "girly," complex theories of gender, social status and communication lie behind what we say, usually without our knowing it. (Barnard, 2007: Introduction)

If we turn to structuralism, the meaning (denotation) of the word "fat" when referencing human beings has the following dictionary definition: "corpulence, obesity or plumpness" (Collins, 2005: 592), which with the exception of "obesity" could be considered facts but also carry within them loaded meanings. In the perceived unpleasantness of Lagerfeld's observation, however, they are certainly meant as an insult because—as Barnard observed—many complex theories come into play and they determine how we interpret it at a cultural (connotative) level. Consequently, given that in our culture, the canonical criterion of feminine beauty—certainly in the world of Lagerfeld—is to be as skinny as possible, to call somebody "fat" is not an attractive option because it does not fulfill the cultural conventions of thinness, which is Lagerfeld's point, although by any other standard Adele is a most attractive woman. As Lagerfeld has a long history as a public figure of calling people "fat," rather than "curvaceous" or another such positive term used within the body activist movement, he links his thought to the general post-1920s obsession with criticizing any woman seen to be "plump" or "corpulent": "While euphemisms may come and go to refer to the fat, female body, fat (like fleshy fat itself) has stubbornly held on over the past century" (communication, Lauren Downing Peters with Peter McNeil, February 21, 2017; Downing Peters ("Fashion Plus" (2016)).

The same analysis is applicable to the second example in which the accusation that clothes belonging to the "controversial" fashion brand American Apparel were "deemed" by "a watchdog" as "overtly sexual." Nothing happens here either: we are simply informed that some clothes have been found to fall short of the moral standards required for public display. It stands to reason that if something is **that** "overtly sexual" as the clothes under discussion, they should never have been allowed to find their way into a shop window in the first place, in order to avoid giving offense.

Randall traces the definition of hard news to 1882, when John B. Bogart, city editor of the *New York Sun* had this to say: "it is not news if a dog bites a man, but it is news if a man bites a dog" (Randall, 2011: 26). Apart from being very funny, this indicates the key characteristics news needs to fulfill in order to be "news worthy." Randall lists "fresh, unpublished, unusual" and of course "generally interesting," and it goes without saying that "man biting dog" is certainly unusual!

Randall also identifies an interesting category within this definition of news—"news fashion" —and this is how he defines it:

There is such a factor as news fashion—subjects which suddenly swim into the news consciousness and are, for a time, flavour of the month. This is seen at its most glaring in the activities which have perhaps been around for a long time in a fairly unobtrusive way, but which suddenly acquire a phrase or word to describe them. (Randall, 2011: 27–8)

Randall traces the history of news fashion to the nineteenth century, when in 1862 *The Times* brought into focus something that was already lurking in people's consciousness—"garotting" (attacks from behind)—by reporting a veritable "epidemy" of the gruesome assaults. An analogous news fashion phenomenon emerged in the United Kingdom in the postwar period, which came to be known as "moral panic," defined by Ian Marsh and Gaynor Melville in their article "Moral Panics and the British Media—a Look at Some Contemporary 'Folk Devils'":

The term moral panic has been widely adopted both by the mass media and in everyday usage to refer to the exaggerated social reactions caused by the activities of particular groups and/or individuals. Such activities are invariably seen (at the time at least) as major social concerns and the media led reaction magnifies and widens the "panic" surrounding them. (Marsh and Melville, 2011)

Its origins have been traced to Stanley Cohen's book *Folk Devils and Moral Panics* of 1964. We can list a multitude of recent examples ranging from drugs to terrorism, but in many instances "moral panic" can be media manipulated for scare mongering and intimidation, which are ultimately immoral practices. Certain "fashion events" such as the extreme meanings (often criminalistic) attributed to the over-the-top "zoot suit" worn by Black American, Mexican American, and Philippine American youth in the 1950s have been uncovered by Kathy Peiss as in part the creation of the media and authorities (Peiss, 2014). Other class-induced examples include the "Teddy Boys in the 1950s," the "Mods and Rockers" in the 1960s, the "punks" of the 1970s, the drug-enhanced "acid house" parties of the 1980s, and the weird phenomenon of "road rage" which appeared in the world press in the 1990s. All of these, with the exception of road rage, were sartorial fashion stories as well.

By way of conclusion we would like to revert to Bradford's section on news and fashion, which is very different from the concept of "news fashion" introduced by Randall, whose more unsavory consequence was the emergence of "moral panic." Bradford gives a couple of examples from *Vogue* (online), one an interview with French actress Marion Cotillard, the other with Donatella Versace. The first one reads "Marion Cotillard's BAFTA [British Academy of Film and Television Awards] red carpet look took just an hour and a half to create" (Alexander, 2013 in Bradford, 2015:112), and in the second example we find Ms Versace expressing her wish to dress the Queen of England in black leather garments (Jones, 2012 in Bradford, 2015:112). To this we can but comment: "we rest our case!"

The feature

What is a fashion feature as opposed to fashion news and how can it be defined? In her book *Fashion Journalism*, Julie Bradford introduced the fashion feature as follows: "Features have been described as the beating heart of a publication, the stories that give it personality, imagination and a voice. Although they are usually topical, features are less tied to the news agenda than news stories, and can explore any topic under the sun so long as it's interesting to the target reader." Moreover, as already pointed out, the word "feature" seems to be regarded as a convenient umbrella term which covers practically everything that is not "news": "On newspapers and magazines, lots of things come under the features remit—not just features themselves, but profiles, listings, reviews, readers' letters, book serialisations, personal columns and agony aunts" (Bradford, 2015: 115). In this sense Bradford concurs with David Randall, who also lists under the heading of "features" the interview, the opinion poll, as well as the review. Regarding fashion features Bradford rightly points out that "what journalists call features proper—generally longer articles exploring an issue or talking point—are in short supply in fashion journalism, in general magazines at least" (Bradford, 2015: 113).

This is significant because as a newcomer to journalism, fashion journalism is still in pursuit of developing its own voice by placing fashion center stage, and secondly, the bulk of fashion writing is magazine rather than newspaper writing that, as a rule, does not go for "features proper." Suffice it to take a look at the top international magazines to see that they are almost written as bullet points or worse still, we find advertorial rather than editorial.

Fortunately this is beginning to change and we selected two publications to make our point: the *Financial Times*—which is yet to be surpassed in terms of quality fashion reporting—and the second from a relatively new magazine whose deceptive glossy look hides an encouraging content, called *Numéro*.

There is no doubt that the *Financial Times* owes its quality fashion reporting to Vanessa Friedman—at present Fashion Director and Chief Fashion Critic for the *New York Times*—who between 2002 and 2014 was fashion editor for the *Financial Times*: she was the first person to acquire the title. We chose a fashion feature entitled "Into the Black" by Mark C. O'Flaherty whose subtitle—"Japanese aesthetics" —reveals its focus, and this has to be fashion journalism at its best.

O'Flaherty covers Rei Kawakubo's spring/summer collection 2010 for *Comme des Garçons* at Paris fashion week 2009. Together with her peers Yohji Yamamoto and Issey Miyake, the Japanese contingent created a revolution in Paris, when they first appeared at the end of the 1970s and they continue to astonish and delight, although they are now regarded as "establishment." The central issue addressed here is "how exactly has the Japanese aesthetic changed what we wear?" and to answer this question, O'Flaherty enlisted the opinion of some of the top fashion personalities, starting with Claire Wilcox:

> When the Japanese arrived in France, western fashion was surprisingly conventional," says Claire Wilcox, fashion curator at the V&A. "They had a huge impact, creating a disruption of construction." By which she means unstructured, deconstructed and skewed garments, acting as the antithesis of an era defined by the sculpted shoulder pad and Alaïa's body-hugging garments. "It's about opposition to body shape," says Wilcox. "A Miyake Pleats Please dress moves in opposition to the natural form and Kawakubo's bumps collection was a total distortion of the human body. (*Financial Times*, October 3/October 4, 2009, 6, Life and Arts)

The subsequent list of interviewees is equally impressive, including Belgian designer Ann Demeulemeester of the "Antwerp Six" fame, British designers Rick Owens and Hussein Chalayan, and Professor Wendy Dagworthy of the Royal College of Art, and they all agree on the radical *volte face* introduced in Western European fashion by Japanese designers.

In 2014, Jo Ellison was appointed as fashion editor of the *Financial Times* to replace Vanessa Friedman, and seven years after Mark C O'Flaherty she reports from Paris fashion week. What we notice is very much a matter of "plus ça change": same issues, same preoccupations, but with different players. While O'Flaherty concentrated on one designer, Rei Kawakubo, through whom he introduced the topic of the new fashion aesthetic introduced by the Japanese in Europe, Ellison covers fashion week in its entirety, sharing with the readers the latest developments and changes at the highest level in the couture world, such as the resignation of Raf Simmons at the house of Dior. Her feature "Couture Club" (*FT Weekend* January 30/January 31, 2016, p. 5) however behaves more like a reportage, which is what she herself calls it in her charmingly alliterative subtitle: "Report: Brash, blushing and all kinds of beautiful—whatever the super rich want to wear, Paris had it made. By Jo Ellison."

She does not start with what is on offer in terms of the latest "look"; instead, she starts with an important piece of news—"business is booming"— and that can only be positive, as confirmed by the *monstre sacré* of *haute couture*, Karl Lagerfeld:

> When asked about sales of Chanel haute couture last year, Karl Lagerfeld, the house's creative director of 33 years said: "Unbelievable. It is incredible how well it's doing."

And after all this, we move to the clothes summed up by Jo Ellison as follows:

> As for the clothes, it was a mixed season, with the aesthetic swinging between elegant restraint and a rather unabashed, brash extravagance; there was no shortage of vulgar gowns. More notable, however, was the shortage in direction, as evidenced by the continued absence of a new creative head at Dior.

But Ellison singled out one exception regarding "perceived sense of direction":

> No such lack of focus at Chanel, where Karl Lagerfeld had taken the themes of ecology and recyclability to create a collection of astonishing ingenuity and refinement. His spare wooden set recalled the chicest bathhouse in Sweden—grass lawn, a simple, slatted central structure, cerulean blue backdrop. Against all expectations, conservation and couture made a beautiful marriage.

An elegant analysis of the "eco-details" of Lagerfeld's craftsmanship culminates with

> an extraordinary bridal ensemble … a long dress worn with a bomber-jacket-cum-opera-coat and train. It looked like an exotic fur. "No tufts of white cotton," said Lagerfeld. Couture cotton wool; I loved it. The

croissant-shaped hairstyles and graphic eye make-up, meanwhile, were a debt to Picasso's *Head of A Woman* (1931) though Lagerfeld had sensibly refrained from mimicking her giant proboscis nose.

Our final example comes from the international glossy fashion magazine entitled *Numéro,* founded in 1998 by Elisabeth Djian, and we found a statement which explains what motivated her to start the magazine we applaud fullheartedly:

> I was bored with magazines that told me how to seduce a man. I wanted to create this magazine for an intelligent, smart woman who wants to read about art, design, music; not about stupidity—creams that take away wrinkles, you know, which is stupid. (Wikipedia)

It worked because the magazine became international, with a Tokyo edition published in 2007, followed by China (2010), Thailand (2012), and Russia (2013). In addition, there is a *Numeró homme,* launched in 2007.

The latest issue, December 2015–January 2016, entitled *Numéro Céleste,* also confirms that Djian has kept her word as proof that fashion magazines need not be trivial or "about stupidity" (although a large number are or have become so); in fact, what she did was even simpler: she merely reverted to the historical tradition of fashion magazine writing which was informed and intellectual and was aimed at an intelligent and educated readership. We need only mention the equally beautiful *Gazette du bon ton* (1912–1925, published in Paris).

Being a "glossy" fashion magazine, advertising is not in short supply, but unlike the case of other "glossies," which consist almost entirely of advertisements and at best "advertorials" (advertisement pretending to be editorial) with proper editorials in short supply or even absent. In Numero the editorial material starts on page 45 (the magazine has 226 pages to include at the end a section in English) with all the key features.

The list of contents starts with *Édito* (signed Babeth Djian, page 45) which provides an explanation regarding the word "céleste" added to the title of this special issue to do with "the kingdom of the heavens," constellations, galaxies and radiant stars, and a constellation of "celebs" to match. But we note a significant difference: we have a new class of "celebs," which include not only supermodels, as in this instance Gigi Hadid (who appears on the cover of the issue), but such "celebs" as architect Rem Koolhaas, *Balmain's* very young designer Olivier Rousteing, and photographer Bettina Rheims, whose career evolved in the most splendidly improbable manner imaginable from photographing striptease artists to being invited in 1995 by the French president Jacques Chirac to document his election and being commissioned to take his official photograph.

The two interviews. The first by Andrew Ayers and Delphine Roche with Rem Koolhaas focused on his collaboration with Miuccia Prada and

Patrizio Bertelli and the second by Philip Utz with Olivier Rousteing, while well documented and serious, are an enjoyable read. But our attention was attracted by a beautifully written (Olivier Joyard) review of the film *Carol* directed by Todd Haynes (Studio Canal/Weinstein, 2015), which tells a story of forbidden lesbian love between a rich woman Carol (played by Cate Blanchett) and a shop assistant (played by Rooney Mara), from which we quote one paragraph:

> Almost inevitably, each shot is veiled in melancholy, as if everything were already over when it had barely begun, as if catastrophe were eroding pleasure at the very moment it was born, as if the present became, in an instant, an inaccessible memory. This Proustian intensification is something we already saw at the beginning of the century with *In the Mood for Love*; while Carol doesn't quite reach the legendary depth of Wong Kar-way's masterpiece—its narrative is more linear for a start—it gets voluptuously close, and leaves a lasting impression on the viewer. (Joyard, 2016: English section, p. 4)

Here we have an example of writing that adds considerably to the experience of watching that fashion-saturated, evocative film.

Finally, we turn to and provide two interrelated examples drawn from Miller's experience as a journalist. During the 1980s and 1990s Miller worked as a freelance journalist both for the national press and specialized art magazines. In 1990, the *Weekend FT* (*Financial Times*, Saturday February 17, 1990) published her piece entitled "The Brechtian Nightmare," a ruminative (the *FT* editor called it "impressionistic") feature about the aftermath of the 1989 Romanian "Revolution," culminating with the capture of President Nicolae Ceausescu and his wife Elena, who were promptly executed by the firing squad on Christmas Day 1989. The bloody event put an end to one of the most brutal Communist regimes in Eastern Europe which lasted twenty-four years. One of the most dramatic *volte face* in the modern history of Romania, this event needed however to be understood within the wider context of the civil unrest in Germany resulting in the "Fall of the Berlin Wall"—(a barrier built between East and West Berlin by the German Democratic Republic in 1961 to separate it from the "corrupt capitalist regime" of Western Germany). On October 3, 1990, Eastern and West Germany were reunited, but it was not until 1992 that the demolition of the wall was completed.

Miller decided to return to Romania to see for herself what was happening and how the people of Bucharest were coping, but beforehand she approached several newspapers in London to ask whether they would be interested to publish some stories. The answer was a resounding "yes!"— which was wonderful because never before, or in fact since, did Miller encounter so much enthusiasm from the press during her freelance career, which fortunately coincided with these events in European history. She was given freehand to choose what she wanted and she did.

Hitherto, Miller worked as an exhibition and book reviewer, mostly for the *Times* and the *Times Higher Education*, and knowing her remit, she never suggested to write anything else. But she could certainly write stories herself, because there were lots of powerful stories to tell from Bucharest. The first example is entitled "The Brechtian Nightmare" (Romanian Sanda Miller reflects on the country since the revolution) (*Weekend FT* (IX)—*Financial Times*, Saturday, February 17, 1990).

Miller here made use of what Sally Adams defines as the "five categories or types of introduction," which in practice could also be combined elements: the "strong/provocative/intriguing statement/narrative/anecdote; description/scene-setting option but in the end/quote" (Adams in Hicks et al., 2008: 54). Decided to let her instinct rule (not sound advice to be offered to an aspiring journalist for the simple reason that it adds to the seemingly nebulous definition of "features"), but she knew what she wanted: she wanted to convey the almost mystical atmosphere which gripped Bucharest during the Christmas of 1989 in the aftermath of the execution of the Ceausescus. And so, she told simply about what she saw in the streets: the white snow, the little ad hoc wooden crosses, and burning candles placed in the most unexpected places in the streets of Bucharest—near trees, by the road side, in front of doors. She told about the people walking, standing, or gathered in groups, as if they had all the time in the world, some were discussing quietly, some demonstrating with placards but judging from the downright childish requests written on them—the actual request was less important than the desire to seem revolutionary and anarchic. In the opening paragraph Miller captured the eerie atmosphere:

A grey February morning in Bucharest and business is as usual: people wrapped up warmly stride purposefully along the boulevards; buses, cars and the occasional lorry speed down busy main roads, contributing to the cacophony of urban noises associated with any metropolis. How deceptive. Soon enough, this impression of normality was dispelled when I came across a kind of makeshift commemorative shrine. Defiantly placed at a major junction between the *Republicii* and *Magheru* boulevards, it consisted of several primitively assembled wooden crosses surrounded by bunches of fresh flowers and candles ... hundreds of thin, yellow-lit candles to which more lit candles were added by a continuous stream of newcomers. They were bringing flowers to those killed on that spot during the revolution. You began to notice more shrines; at street corners, in the middle of squares or on pavements hugging the walls covered with slogans and graffiti against the defunct Ceausescu regime.

The next stage she embarked upon is content, and Adams gives the following advice:

Ways to write feature body copy are many, various and determined by the brief. All should include good, clear, lively writing whatever the subject and whatever the aim—information, description, anecdotes, quotes, comment, analysis. (Adams in Hicks et al., 2008: 62)

Miller had no brief, but she wanted to capture a moment in time, to tell the readers "how it was" or rather what was it like to be in Bucharest in the winter of 1990.

After the introduction, how did she structure the feature? She did not! It structured her; she simply became a Baudelarian *flâneur* wandering the streets and letting things happen. How beautifully does Baudelaire put this in his seminal "Salon" review dedicated to the illustrator Constantin Guys, the essay better known as "The Painter of Modern Life":

> The crowd is his domain, just as the air is the bird's, and water that of the fish. His passion and his profession is to merge with the crowd. For the perfect idler, for the passionate observer it becomes an immense source of enjoyment to establish his dwelling in the throng, in the ebb and flow, the bustle, the fleeting and the infinite ... The observer is a prince enjoying his incognito wherever he goes. (Baudelaire (1863) 1972: 399–400)

With hindsight, the trope Miller instinctively adopted was that of the Baudelarian wanderer who mingled and observed—and there was much to be observed!

Her next encounter approximated a Dada event, and that ought not to come as a surprise, given that Romania is the country of origin of the most anarchic French avant-garde movement, Dadaism, with one of its main founders, Tristan Tzara, being Romanian:

> In front of the National Theatre, people were congregating in separate groups. Hyde Park Corner in the middle of Bucharest. The crowd made way until I reached the middle of one group but what I saw was not some orator but a silent protestor. The placard around his neck announced that he was on hunger strike for free television.

Free television? A woman scurried by shouting with disdain: *Si tot crapam de foame* (we are still dying of hunger). Unexpectedly, the protester called Miller's name, and underneath the black woollen hat, pulled down to the eyebrows, she recognized the son of one of her friends from high school, Rodica Dumitrescu, who became a top political journalist writing for the magazine *Lumea* (*The World*)—a kind of Romanian *Time* magazine— one of the speakers in the adjacent crowd. She had interrupted her stay in Warsaw and returned to Bucharest alerted by the possibility of civil war. It sounded so portentous that Miller burst into laughter, but her school friend was in no laughing mood and had little time to explain.

What brought the feature to life was Miller's interaction with witnesses, but unlike in a news report when they are only expected to confirm what happened, in a feature, it is their opinions that matter. She talked to a theatre student, Despina Marian, and an architect, Vlad Barbu, and what she learnt confirmed the uncanny experience:

> The revolution was so unexpected that everything we are experiencing seems unreal. I would not be surprised to switch on my TV set and see Ceausescu preaching his usual inanities—that we must fight for disarmament, peace, etc … Too many unexpected phenomena are happening and we cannot cope.

But there was some progress, however modest, especially noticeable in shop windows; when Miller visited Romania for a study trip, in the summer of 1989 she noticed with dismay how empty the supermarkets were: apart from bottles of undrinkable Romanian champagne, tinned green peas and something which looked like shredded cabbage in pickle jars. Now only six months later, the shop windows and the supermarket shelves looked almost joyful:

> I saw in a window of a supermarket bunches of fresh kohlrabi. For me the ridiculous vegetable became almost a symbolic harbinger of a Romanian spring. In front of a bakery, boxes full of freshly baked bread unloaded from a lorry filled the air with the reassuring smell of normality but, paradoxically, this only seemed to add to the surrealist effect of dislocation I have been experiencing.

Later that evening Miller had dinner at the flat of her hosts—Professor Raoul Sorban, his theatre costume designer wife Eva, and their teenage daughter—in a haven of normality. But they were brought back to reality by the TV news which broadcasted the end of the trial of the "infamous four": Ceausescu's ministers, Manea Manescu, Tudor Postelnicu, Emil Bobu, and Ion Dinca; they were all jailed for life; there was more to come:

> This was followed by the trial of Elena Barbulescu—sister of the former dictator. Dressed like a peasant, she refused to utter a single word. She stood alone in the middle of the room. We could only hear the voices of her interrogators.

It was uncomfortable, bizarre, and everything appeared so unreal, as if it were a play.

> Suddenly it seemed that we were watching a Brecht play. I could almost hear the insidious: "Oh, moon of Alabama/we now must say good-bye/ we've lost our good old mamma … Mahagonny." Bucharest was the socialist Mahagonny, only the nightmare was real. Frighteningly, it is not over yet.

The second feature Miller wrote for the newspaper *Observer* (Sunday April 1, 1990, p. 57) was entitled "The consolation of beauty" and its subtitle was "Sanda Miller, just back from a trip to Bucharest, met the beauty team at Romania's largest cosmetic institute." This was a much more matter-of-fact feature for which Miller had a vague brief from her editor: to talk to the beauty team which consisted of three very special and brave women—Cornelia Cochilie, Liliana Pasca, and Adriana Ioanes.

This was a special feature because it was based on the testimony of the three women interviewed by Miller, but its theme was the everyday life of three professional women during Ceausescu's regime. Like the vast majority of women in former communist Romania, the three beauticians worked full time while managing their roles as wives and mothers, and each interviewee had a story to tell (Figure 6.1):

> Cornelia Cochilie, the most talkative was a vivacious 44 year old blonde with lovely eyes and a perfect skin. Married but childless, she has her own

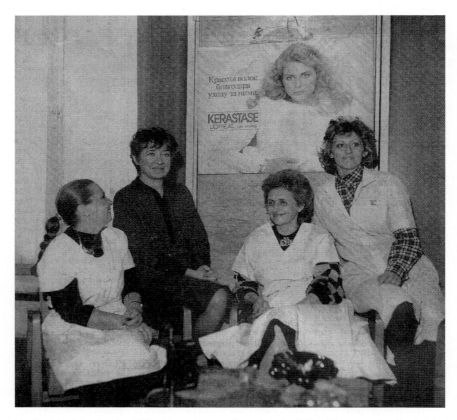

FIGURE 6.1 *Sanda Miller interviewing Cornelia Cochilie*, Observer, *April 1, 1990. Author's Collection/Photographer Ion Milea.*

parents and those of her husband, who is an engineer, to take care of. Her mother has had two brain operations and Cornelia took a month's unpaid leave to be with her in hospital. "I understood then for the first time the depths of human misery, when I saw people who had just undergone brain surgery being kept in unheated rooms." Although their joint income is well above average, Cornelia and her husband are unable to save or to have a holiday abroad. They own their car (bought on HP), their clothes are ordinary, their two-roomed apartment is ordinary, their everyday life is ordinary: a basic sort of existence in which there is no space for any luxuries.

Liliana Pasca's story was not that different from that of her colleague:

> Liliana Pasca the most senior of the team belongs to the first generation of professionally-trained beauticians in Romania, who graduated from the *Scoala Technica Sanitara* between 1965 and 1967. Liliana's generation had more thorough training than that of her 21-year-old daughter, Christiana, who is also a beautician. "I managed to survive because I am a trained laboratory technician and was always able to make my own products, such as a tonic lotion or a cream, none of which was available. Make-up is not compulsory for every beautician, but I am passionate about it. It is spectacular and glamorous and gives immediate satisfaction, while cosmetic treatment, which is curative, is a long-term affair."

Miller asked her to describe an ordinary working day and was humbled into silence:

> I get up at about 4.30 am to cook hot food for my family because we only have gas at night. Then I come to work and often I have to drink a lot of coffee to keep going. After finishing here I go to my technical college where I teach make-up. Sometimes I take off my shoes because my feet are too swollen. When I get home I do my ironing or washing. Our Sundays, in fact the Sunday of every woman in Romania, means only one thing—housework.

The youngest of the group, Adriana Ioanes, was a make-up specialist. She was divorced and had a nine-year-old son and she also represented the team of the Institute at international make-up competitions, which meant strictly the USSR and the satellite countries, but even among Eastern Europeans she was unable to compete because of lack of materials and information, and for that reason in 1988 she decided to stop competing:

> I felt so unhappy in Poland, for instance, when I saw the kinds of make-up the Russians or the Poles worked with, while our team turned up with all sorts of leftovers and had to improvise.

But it was something else which brought tears into Miller's eyes: the optimism and joy with which these hardworking women were looking toward their future, in a country now freed of the oppressive Ceausescu regime. This is what they said:

> You must know that our women here are honest and hardworking and with all these new perspectives opening up, we have high hopes, very high hopes indeed. In fact we are in a hurry to begin to do things.

In conclusion, fashion features are an important space for thinking through fashion. They do not have to be based on the idea of the sole creative individual (the designer), or the cost of handbags, or whether French women look more chic. There is a great deal of potential for expanding and explaining what fashion means to people who are not its cognsocenti, and indeed they too can have their perspectives on fashion expanded by good journalism. In journalism the feature is such an all-inclusive category (as we already pointed out elsewhere) that in some accounts it gobbles up everything in its way, with the exceptions of the high-brow "hard news." But even here we can encounter, according to David Randall (2011: 219), problems, because to try and distinguish between news writing and feature writing is a matter of semantics, e.g. tantamount (as Randall puts it) with "hair splitting debates." That is followed by his generous list (pp. 220–1) we reproduced in the introduction of various categories of features, ranging from the well-known "fly on the wall" approach to "vox pops" to which we can add "profiles," "interviews," and "reviews," which we consider to belong elsewhere! Therefore, for the sake of argument, let's just say that a piece of writing which is not straight news, straight poetry, Plato's dialogues or Marcel Proust's "Remembrance of Things Past" can alternatively be called a "feature"!

The interview and profile

What is an interview?

Interviewing is a tool of the trade but the interview is not! The interview is one of the main categories or type of journalism based on a "Question and Answer" technique that is defined in the dictionary as "a conversation with or questioning of a person, usually conducted for television, radio, or a newspaper" (Collins, 2005: 848).

As pointed out in our Introduction, the interview is technically a dialogue rather than a conversation, the only difference between them being their final cause (*telos*), which in the first instance can be summed up as an exchange, although it can also be a questioning, while in the latter, the relationship is altered in as much as the interviewer is also the questioner aiming to uncover something about the interviewee.

We can even introduce a third category that is neither dialogue nor interview but something in-between, and the example comes from Lewis Carroll's celebrated book *Alice in Wonderland* (1865):

> Who are you? said the Caterpillar.
> This was not an encouraging opening for a conversation. Alice replied, rather shyly, "I—I hardly know, sir, just at present—at least I know who I was when I got up this morning, but I think I must have been changed several times since then."
> "What do you mean by that?" said the Caterpillar sternly. "Explain yourself!"…
> "I'm afraid I can't put it more clearly," Alice replied very politely, "for I can't understand it myself to begin with; and being so many different sizes in a day is very confusing." (See: The Philosopher's Alice: Alice's adventures in wonderland and through the looking-glass by Lewis Carroll, St. Martin's Press, 1974)

Hitherto, most books dealing with journalism and its individual categories provide practical advice about how to research, plan, and conduct an interview as well as the most important "do's" and "don'ts" to be incorporated or avoided by the interviewer. This type of approach is based on practical experience, but as it has repeatedly been pointed out, although the questions can be selected beforehand, the main pitfall when conducting an interview is its unpredictable outcome—as any practicing journalist can confirm.

The reason is simple: while the questions can be rigorously prepared beforehand, this is not the case with the answers, which can be unpredictable in the extreme:

> Interviews, whether in person or over the telephone are not scripted and you should be prepared for unexpected answers, to follow their implications and ask follow-up questions. They will often be long pedantic affairs, as you persist with a question you want answered or something you want to understand. They are not opportunities for you to tell that official what you think of him, show off your knowledge or engage your subject in heated debate. (Randall, 2011: 73)

This may call for a very special person to be the interviewer and the question to be asked then is: who would make such an ideal interviewer? What kind of journalist would be fit for purpose? According to Sally Adams and Wynford Hicks, authors of the book *Interviewing for Journalists*, the most useful *characteristic* with regard to the personal *attributes* of the good interviewer are *likeability, charm*, and *curiosity*, and Adams and Wynford should know, given that they are both seasoned journalists.

The most useful characteristic for an all-round interviewer is to be likeable, the sort of person who can get on with almost anybody and is interested in everybody: a person who people are happy to talk to, who comes across as a human being first, a journalist second. The most valuable attribute is probably curiosity, followed by charm, keen powers of observation, doggedness, flexibility and fairness. Then add the ability to think fast, analyse, keep a poker face when necessary, a broad general knowledge and plenty of scepticism. (Adams and Hicks, 2009:: 5)

What is a profile?

As pointed out in our Introduction, for some reason the profile appears as a kind of *Cinderella* among the categories of journalism because it tends to be overlooked or simply passed over in silence, and one of the reasons for this may well be that it sits in between interviewing and features. No wonder David Randall considers the profile to be a feature:

> Normally a study of personality at the centre of a story, but it can also be the portrait of a place, organisation, religion, etc. It can be a report of one encounter with the subject, or gather many views and give a rounded portrait. (Randall, 2011: 221)

The profile does not fare better with the duo Adams and Hicks. Thus, in *Interviewing for Journalists*, we have the fact that almost every newspaper or magazine Q & A feature has some questions that can be used for a general profile interview (Adams and Hicks, 2009: 58), and in *Writing for Journalists* it only makes an appearance in the "Glossary of terms used in journalism" (pp. 171–82) as follows: "profile in words of individual or organisation" (Adams and Hicks, 2008: 179).

The prestigious "School of Journalism and Communication" (University of Oregon) includes an online teaching module "Media Writing; unit J206" with examples of profiles written by their students, and what strikes the reader is the variety of subject matter, including "Profile of a Symphony Conductor"; "Profile of a 'Hash House Harrier'" (to you and me these are international groups of non-competitive running school clubs), and "Profile of Don Bolles, Arizona Republic investigative reporter," which won the first place in the national Hearst student journalism awards profile categories, 2007.

We do have an admirable example of profile writing in the UK *Financial Times*: "Lunch with the FT" and publication of a book entitled "Lunch with the FT: 52 Classic Interviews" by Lionel Barber (2015) which testifies to its success. These pieces are also given pride of place on page 3 in the main section of the *Financial Times*. A cursory look at examples of "celebs" we kept on file published between 2013 and 2016 reveals a wonderful and quite idiosyncratic set of choices. In many cases the reaction of the reader would be "who?," which is understandable, because typically the *FT* would choose the real power moguls instead of the "glitterati"!.

Historical overview

While it is generally accepted that the interview is regarded "as the central activity in modern journalism," there seems to be little exact information about when and how the interview emerged as an independent category to take center stage in the practice of journalism. According to one account however, the interview arrived in Britain from the United States toward the end of the nineteenth century, and for that reason it is reasonable to assume that it originated in the American press:

> According to Christopher Silvester, the interview came to Britain from the United States towards the end of the nineteenth century. It was part of the "new journalism" that turned the media world upside down. From a stuffy, pompous thing that could interest only a minority of the serious-minded, journalism became a lively means of informing and entertaining millions of people. (Adams with Hicks, 2009: Introduction)

In the above quote we have a seminal example of how researchers and academics qualify their statements by supporting them with the voice of authority. For the historian of art or dress this is a straightforward matter and a part of undergraduate training: any historian relies on primary sources—be they visual or written—such as texts, objects, or works of art, and in the case of the latter, also material evidence (e.g., historic dress and other such material culture).

In an instance such as the one referenced above, the situation is less clear-cut and therefore open to debate. Of course, issues such as interpretation are crucial in the way the historian extracts meaning from existing primary sources which are also silent sources, but in the case of journalism what could count as a primary and therefore authoritative source?

In this example, we will have to justify the choice of Christopher Silvester as an authoritative source to start with, and if the result is satisfactory we will accept that the interview originated in the American press during the nineteenth century.

We start by investigating our proposed authoritative source: Christopher Silvester. Christopher Silvester is a British, Cambridge-educated journalist, whose work *Penguin Book of Interviews: An Anthology from 1859 to the Present Day*, published in 1993, conveys upon him a status that is authoritative. Moreover, Adams and Hicks argue:

[T]he interview was part of the "new journalism" that turned the media world upside down. From a stuffy, pompous thing that could interest only a minority of the serious-minded, journalism became a lively means of informing and entertaining millions of people. (Adams and Hicks, 2009: 1)

In addition to the introduction, their book is divided into eleven chapters, each dealing with a specific aspect of the interview, starting with research, inception, and techniques, and although the book concentrates on the print aspect, other media, such as "Interviewing for the Internet": (Chapter 8), are also dealt with. Another important aspect that they address is that of the interviewee, where good advice is on offer, as in "Interviewing Politicians": (Chapter 9) and "Interviewing Celebrities" (Chapter 10). Practical advice is on offer in the case of difficult interviewees who are the main cause of the unpredictability of the outcome of an interview: "Challenging Interviewees": (Chapter 11). In this category the authors list: "reluctant interviewees, inexperienced interviewees, business people, vulnerable people, children and the bereaved" ("death knocks" and "fatals" in newspaper jargon singled out all require special handling, as do interviews where PR's sit in on the interview, and what's called "two-banders," where it's the interviewers who double up) (Adams and Hicks, 2009: 165).

The interview as dialogue

If we accept that the interview is based on a "question and answer" technique, then the interview falls under the wider category of the dialogue, the time honored way of uncovering information by asking questions and giving answers which can be traced back to antiquity, specifically ancient Greece, where it was widely used in many systems of communication, such as the theatre. The very idea of classifying the theatre as a system of communication may appear strange to say the least, but "live theatre was both the original mass medium and the first multimedia experience" and regarded as "the first communications medium to persuade an audience to part with money to watch it" (Parry, 2011: 42–3). Its most important aspect, however, is its form, given that the theatre stems from the Dionysian festivals in dialogue form:

Dionysus, the Greek god of fertility, was the patron of vineyards and wine ... a major annual festival was held in his honour. At this event a chorus of about 50 people sang and chanted ... These performances became organised competitions—the *American Idol* of ancient Athens. At some point they started to feature a single performer who would stand in front of the chorus and recite solo verse. In 534 BC one of these competitive events was won by a priest or "actor" called Thespis. The concept of the theatre and the profession of thespian were, allegedly, born in that year. (Parry, 2011: 44)

The origins of the theatre are to be found in the *dithyramb* (unison hymn) sung in honor of Dionysus, the god of wine. In the earliest plays, the main protagonist was the *chorus* formed of fifty members who performed around the altar of Dionysus that was placed in the center of the stage. Initially, the *dithyramb*, whose initial function was to tell of the life and deeds of Dionysus, widened to include "tales of demi-gods or heroes, legendary ancestors of the Greeks and their associate peoples" (Hartnoll, 1985: 8–9). But Thespis changed all that: "The great innovation that Thespis made was to detach himself from the chorus and, in the person of the god or hero whose deeds were being celebrated, to engage in dialogue with it" (Hartnoll, 1985: 10). This is how dialogue was first introduced in the theatre, and it became the dominant form still employed today, whether in plays written for the stage or to be read.

Nor was the theatre the only medium structured as dialogue; we find it (unexpectedly) in philosophy. Even for people not versed in it, many know about Plato's *Dialogues*, written in 399 BCE (the year of Socrates's death), with his last "Laws" left unpublished at his death in 347 BCE. It would therefore be useful to offer a definition of the **dialogue**. Collins offers six definitions, all of which amount to the same essential characteristic—an exchange:

A dialogue then is defined as a "conversation between two or more people; an exchange of opinions on a particular subject, discussion; the lines spoken by characters in drama or fiction; a particular passage of conversation in a literary or dramatic work; a literary composition in the form of dialogue; a political discussion between representatives of two nations or groups." (Collins, 2005: 457)

The Greek fifth century BCE philosopher Plato (428–347 BCE) left us a legacy that includes thirty-five dialogues as well as well as thirteen letters (epistles) also ascribed to him (Cooper [Plato] 1997: Introduction, IX). What makes Plato's philosophical writings so special is that he wrote them in dialogue form, and we ask ourselves what was the reason behind it?

Why did Plato write dialogues? What does it mean for the reader of his works that they take this form? Philosophers of earlier generations expounded their views and developed their arguments either in the meters of epic poetry ... or in short prose writings or collections of remarks ... or in rhetorical display pieces ... Socrates himself, of course, was not a writer at all but engaged in philosophy only orally, in face-to-face question-and-answer discussions ... the dialogue form for philosophical writing began within the circle of those for whom philosophy meant in the first instance the sort of inquiry Socrates was engaged in. (Cooper [Plato] 1997: Introduction: XVIII)

Philosophy, then, began as a "face-to-face question-and-answer discussion," and if we return to the opening lines of this chapter, the interview is a technique based on the very same principles—"question and answer"—in both instances aimed at uncovering, whether a deeper understanding of ethical, epistemological, or metaphysical problems found in philosophy or at a simpler level, information about the interviewee. How incredible that the sensationalist interviews conducted by a current affairs anchor-person or Oprah Winfrey have their origins in a form that most people would have thought antithetical.

By way of example regarding the Platonic use of dialogue, are the three dialogues that relate the trial and execution of Socrates by the Athenians in 399 BC on grounds of "impiety" for offending the Olympian gods. The basis for this accusation was his *philosophi*. The first one, "Apology" (defense speech) of Socrates aged seventy, was made in front of the jury consisting of 501 male Athenians, but Socrates refused to comply with their requirements and was condemned to death. In the second, entitled "Crito," Socrates refused yet again to be saved by his friend Crito, who offered to bribe the jailers and help him escape from Athens. But the most touching of them is "Phaedo," which is about Socrates's last hours and his death in jail, and the very last exchange between Socrates and Crito as he was dying, having been made to swallow poison. It brought tears not only to the eyes of his friends and even the jailer, but they continue to bring tears into our eyes, more than two millennia later:

> As his belly was getting cold Socrates uncovered his head—he had covered it—and said—these were his last words—"Crito, we owe a cock to Asclepius; make this offering to him and do not forget"; "It shall be done," said Crito, "tell us if there is anything else" ... Shortly afterwards Socrates made a movement; the man uncovered him and his eyes were fixed. Seeing this Crito closed his mouth and his eyes. Such was the end of our comrade, Echecrates ... of all those we have known the best, and also the wisest and the most upright. (Cooper [Plato]1997: 100)

The subsequent history of the dialogue from the Antiquity to our times testifies to its endurance as a technique employed in a variety of contexts, each with its specific ways of using question and answer as the basis on which a written text—be that either philosophical or literary text—is present to the readers, but most importantly, how the "dialogue" became the "interview," and according to Christopher Silvester, took center stage within the practice of journalists.

How to interview?

Sally Adams and Wynford Hicks's book *Interviewing for Journalists,* based on the practical knowledge of the authors, constitutes a solid basis for learning the "tools of the trade" to which each journalist will of course add their own experience, point of view, and personal approach in conducting an interview for the press. Adams and Hicks start with what they call the basics as applied to news interviewing, which consists of the "famous" six questions journalists adopted as the "mantra" of their trade. These are easy to remember and they are simply **who, what, when, where, why,** and **how.** Thus, if a journalist covers a town planning argument for a weekly newspaper, they need to know the following:

- **Who** are the individuals, company or organization seeking planning permission, and who are those protesting against it?
- **What** does the planning application entail? Is it a school, shopping center, luxury block of flats?
- **When** are the key dates? When was the application submitted, for example, and when is the next meeting to discuss it?
- **Why** are protesters so unhappy about it? Why do supporters think it should go ahead? You will need to speak to representatives from both sides to report their view
- **How** are protesters planning to show their disapproval? How are supporters hoping to convince the community that the planning application should go ahead? (Adams and Hicks, 2009: 11).

The same six questions already discussed in our previous chapters are listed by David Randall in his seminal book *The Universal Journalist* (1996), where he links their use to the need for "precision" in journalism and for that reason they are recommended to be asked by the reporter:

- **What?**—What has happened?
- **Who?**—Who has it happened to? Who has done it? Age, appearance, position, Credentials, and any relevant background.
- **Where?**—Where did it happen?
- **When?**—When did it happen? What time, day, month?
- **How?**—How did it happen? Explanations.
- **Why?**—Why did it happen? (Randall, 2011: 169)

These six questions are the basic tools used in interviews in the section on "Categories and categorising" (Adams and Hicks, 2009: 47–52). Adams and Hicks list three recognized main categories: "closed, open and leading," and in the subsequent examples we note that our six essential questions constitute the dominant ones, as we will notice with the example of their "closed questions" recommended for "establishing essentials—names, job titles, locations":

"Did you see the accident?"
"No"

"What's the group's full title?"
"The United Bellringers of Scourie."
"How many boats can moor at the Marina?"
"120."
"What's her middle name?"
"Arabella."
"Where was the last AGM held?"
                              "Birmingham" (Adams and Hicks, 2009: 47)

Chapters 3–7 deal with a comprehensive guideline that will help the aspiring journalist to prepare and conduct an interview. They start with Chapter 3: "Preparing for Interviews," either face-to-face or by telephone, and proceed through to Chapter 4, "Interviewing Techniques," which is the most important, in as much as it deals with the technique of conducting an interview (we shall return to that later), then Chapter 5: "Understanding Interviewees and Avoiding Problems," followed by Chapter 6, "Quotes and Checking Your Information," and finally chapter 7, "Note-Taking and Recording." As mentioned elsewhere, Chapters 9–11 switch from advice for the interviewer to focusing on the different types of interviewees—celebrities, politicians, and especially difficult, awkward, or rude interviewees, and how best to deal with them in a professional manner.

David Randall introduces an important point regarding the various categories (types) of journalism, e.g., news reporting, features, interviews, profiles, by pointing out that these distinctions are by no means clear-cut; in fact, the opposite is the case because he considers that employing techniques associated with a specific category (news) to another (features) could benefit both. Moreover, he suggests that **reporting** should be the generic category that covers the whole lot:

> The truth is that trying to make distinctions between news and features does not get us very far … It produces narrow thinking which can restrict coverage of news to conventional subjects and puts writing it into the unimaginative straitjacket of a formula … Most news pages could benefit from a greater sense of adventure … Similarly, most features sections cry out for sharper research and less indulgent writing. There is no great divide between news and features. Best to think of it all as **reporting.** (Randall, 2011: 219–20)

Among the different approaches listed by Randall in reporting we find the interview:

> Can be either written as a story, with context, background and comments, or given as a verbatim, but edited, account of the interview. If the latter, the questions should not be too long, should be more carefully phrased than usual and any editing of the answers should be made clear with

elipses (...). The subject needs to speak well and interestingly, as there is no scope for making good this deficiency with entertaining commentary from the interviewer. (Randall, 2011: 221)

Case studies of interviews and profiles

We will now offer several examples or "case studies" of interviews as well as profiles, selected from a variety of sources or from our personal experience.

Case study 1. Interview with the music star Madonna by the Hungarian magazine Blikk, as found in Adams and Hicks

We start with a spectacular example published in Adams and Hicks's Appendix 2 entitled "Madonna interviewed as never before" (Adams and Hicks, 2009: 209–10). This interview took place in 1996, when Madonna was interviewed in Hungarian, and the interview translated back into English was reproduced in *Time* magazine. The interview was also reproduced in the *Evening Standard* (August 14, 1996), but the extracts reproduced in the appendix were "plucked from cyberspace":

> **Blikk:** Madonna, Budapest says hello with arms that are spread-eagled. Did you have a visit here that was agreeable? Are you in good odour?...
>
> **Madonna:** Thank you for saying these compliments (holds up hands). Please stop with taking sensationalist photographs until I have removed my garments for all the world to see (laughs). This is a joke I have made.
>
> **Blikk:** Madonna, let's cut toward the hunt. Are you a bold hussy-woman that feasts on men who are tops?
>
> **Madonna:** Yes, yes this is certainly something that brings to the surface my longings...

(Adams and Hicks, 2009: 209–10)

Case study 2. Examples from the press

The use of the interview in dialogue form is not a common occurrence in newspapers; rather, we find them in magazines where space does not come at such a premium. Instead of the "question and answer" form, newspapers prefer to publish the interview as a profile, and one of the most successful examples is the weekly regular interview: "Lunch with the FT" (*Financial Times*, UK). The impressive list of the interviewees includes men and women from all walks of life, of all ages, and from every country and continent on planet Earth, but what links them together is a special attribute: "power," but we are not discussing power of the kind we measure celebrity status or wealth with, but a very different power to do with influencing people, such as that of the German Chancellor Angela Merkel or the Hungarian-born billionaire financier George Soros.

We shall use a very recent profile in the series "Lunch with the FT" as case study.

In the November 5–6, 2016, issue of the *FT* in the *FT* Weekend section (p. 5) *FT*'s current fashion editor interviews Tom Ford: "Lunch with the FT Tom Ford" introducing him as follows to her readership: "Fashion genius, billion dollar businessman, Oscar winning film-maker?" 'I usually do exactly what I say I'm going to do'," the designer tells *Jo Ellison* over steak frites on Mayfair. The venue in question—34 Mayfair—a steak and seafood restaurant on the corner of Grosvenor Square, London where the great man was expecting his interviewer:

> He looks as suave and impeccable as the posters on which he promotes his products. Now 55, the close crop of ebony-coloured hair is flacked with few greys, the 72 hour stubble is not a minute overgrown. His black Tom Ford suit, white shirt and black tie, fastened with a gold pin at the neck, are pristine.

Indeed, this is how he looked and readers find confirmation in the very imposing portrait drawing signed "Ferguson" placed in the middle of the page so that nobody can miss him!

Following the standard *FT* profile pattern, Ellison presents a chronological account of Ford's career starting with his years spent at Gucci, where he arrived in 1990 when the company was about to file for bankruptcy. So successful was he that fourteen years later the company was worth ten billion dollars. But Ford's departure was far from smooth:

> When he left, 14 years later, in the murky wake of the Pinault family buyout, he had risen to become the group's creative director and transformed Gucci into an $10bn luxury conglomerate, incorporating Saint Laurent and Alexander McQueen, among others, with an influence to rival LVMH. He left with $250m in stock options and a bucket full of ire.

Now all this is left unexplained and we suspect that either Ellison assumed that the story is too familiar to be referenced here or maybe at Tom Ford's request. Fact is that this crucial moment in his career is left uncommented.

We proceed to the next important stage of his career in 2009 when he turned to the cinema and released his debut movie—*A Single Man*—with Colin Firth in the main role for which he received a BAFTA. This provides also an opportune moment to reference his forthcoming film *Nocturnal*

Animals, which "was awarded the Grand Jury Prize at the Venice Film Festival" with Amy Adams in the lead as Susan Morrow, a

> successful art gallerist trapped in a superficially perfect career, home and marriage, who is shaken from her emotional analgesia by the arrival of a manuscript, dedicated to her and written by her first husband Edward Sheffield (Jake Gyllenhaal).

The morale of the story being, you cannot have it all!

The interviewer than proceeds to discuss the delicate issue of aging, although at fifty-five years of age Tom Ford has little reason to worry, yet he does and consequently he confessed to surrounding himself with "pictures of Georgia O'Keefe all over my house so I can start to embrace age. Now that I am moving towards 60, I need to start demanding less of what I look like."

We beg to differ Mr. Ford, your grooming reveals a level of perfection not seen since George 'Beau' Brummell achieved the accolade of dandy. But there is little doubt that in 2016 there would be little time for somebody as busy to dedicate so much time to grooming but it is interesting to learn what he had to say about this topic:

> In times past, Ford kept a vice-like grip on any signs of creeping decrepitude. He was once an unusually vocal advocate for Botox. today not so much. "See, I can move my forehead," he says waggling eyebrows that do appear to enjoy a modicum of independent movement. "I watch what I eat, I exercise" … "But I don't ever want to look silly. I sort of like to think of it as looking Best in Class. I'm 55, so let's look good at 55 as you can look. But I'm not trying to look 40, or 30. It's not attainable."

Over steak and frites which just arrived (a special indulgence perhaps), Tom Ford continues on an important topic to do with the way old age is viewed in Western culture and perhaps we have a debt to the United States in this respect, as creators of the cult of youth!

"I think there's a certain beauty that comes with adults that maybe we don't admire or respect enough in our culture," he continues as he picks through the chips. "Louise Nevelson, the artist, was great looking. Really wrinkled, she had that look and dark eyes, and she kept it right up until the end." I suspect the secret to this kind of beauty is to stay very skinny. Skinny enough to slip into a slinky Tom Ford dress. Ford agrees. "Stay thin and stay limber. Do yoga."

But the most important things, including his parenthood, not touching alcohol for seven years and being in therapy, he feels everybody over the age of fifty should make use of, as well as his marriage to Richard Buckley (his husband) whom he met when he was twenty-five years old, are discussed. Although successful, rich, handsome, and in a happy relationship, Tom Ford is far from being the contented person most people would think he ought to be because the story with Gucci still looms large in his psyche, tactfully summed up by Ellison:

> Ford still bears the scars of those months after Gucci when he was engulfed with depression. "I had no voice in contemporary culture," he says of that time. "I had such a powerful voice in the 90s and an identity that I worked very hard to achieve..."

At Ellison's objection (and most of us would support that) he made possibly the strongest remark in the interview: "Fashion is evil," he replies. "You stay out for very long and people forget who you are. And your name loses power." This may well be a clear case of hubris, from his part, but we do see that it is tinged with sadness and regrets at how things evolved in his career in the fashion world.

But the best question Jo Ellison had up her sleeve was left for the end:

> I wonder whether, as the man who helped build the Gucci conglomerate, he doesn't feel partially responsible for the corporate climate, where designers are sacked at will and contracts rarely renewed. Didn't he help usher in this new era of gracelessness?

This is as good as it gets, but of course, it was denied: "It wasn't like that," he insists. "The way we were able to acquire those brands is that I went to each of them and said: "We're buying you because we believe in you, and we're not going to bother you." ... "Which is why, actually I think I'm good with actors, because I know you can't breathe down their neck. They all want to give the best performance, so it's your job to give them the space to do that." The discussion was left at that and what followed more or less exonerated him from such accusations, be they real or putative. Would it not be ironic, Jo Ellison wondered, if he will be remembered in culture as a film maker rather than fashion designer? Or even both, we hasten to add!

Case study 3: Examples from our personal experience as interviewers: Miller with Ionesco

During the 1980s and 1990s Miller worked in journalism on a freelance basis, and wrote both for the national press including *The Times*, *The Financial Times*, *The Sunday Times*, *The Observer*, *The Times Higher Education Supplement*, as well as some of the best-known international art magazines, among them *Artforum* (USA), *The Burlington Magazine*, *Apollo* (UK), *The Irish Art Review* (Ireland), and *Art Press* (France). Miller was fortunate to obtain an interview with the celebrated French-based, Romanian-born, playwright Eugène Ionesco, whose plays such as *The Bald Primadonna* and *The Lesson* and above all *Rhinoceros* became the best known and loved plays in the repertory of the "theatre of the absurd," a new genre which emerged in the 1950s with the writings of Eugène Ionesco, Samuel Beckett, Jean Genet, and Harold Pinter.

Martin Esslin, the acknowledged authority on "the theatre of the absurd," who published his seminal book *The Theatre of the Absurd* (1960) made a distinction between different categories of theatre, distinguishing naturalist theatre, Bertolt Brecht's epic theatre, and it was Esslin who coined the term "The theatre of the absurd," which took its queue from the "world of fantasy and dream." Esslin chose the uncanny play entitled *Amédée* by way of example; in it a married couple are terrified because there is a corpse in the next room:

> perhaps that of the wife's lover killed by the husband, and the corpse keeps growing ... an absurd concept, a growing corpse, but terrifying. It grows so large that finally a huge foot breaks through the door and as it keeps growing gradually pushes the couple out of their house ... a real nightmare but also a powerful image, which on reflection makes sense ... So in plays such as these, the nightmare or dream images also become poetic metaphors of reality. (Esslin, 1983: 65)

Ionesco himself rejected the label "absurd" predicated by Esslin of his plays, but the latter in turn offered an explanation as to why he created it: to help critics and journalists:

> When I wrote my book on the Theatre of the Absurd I tried to provide some sort of help to critics who, I felt, were missing the point of a number of plays I had greatly enjoyed and admired. I tried to isolate and analyse what the plays of Beckett, Ionesco, Adamov, Genet, Pinter, etc, had in common—features such as the absence of a full exposition or solution, a wide use of dreamlike images and situations, a new kind of associative rather than rational logic and so on. (Esslin, 1983: 58–9)

Miller was commissioned to interview Eugène Ionesco and write a feature for *The Sunday Times* in 1985 and so she set off to Paris to meet the playwright, who was living with his wife Rodica in an apartment above the iconic brasserie *La Coupole* on boulevard Montparnasse. After several days of visiting him and being unceremoniously sent away she put all her hopes on the last day of her stay in Paris: October 13, 1985 (which also happened to be her birthday). She decided to take a stance but did not quite know how—What to do? Ionesco was waiting and on this occasion he gave her time to set up the very complicated tape recorder she had borrowed from a radio journalist friend. They started a conversation in Romanian, and at some point he said "I am stuck; do you mind if I will write down some ideas and send them to you by post?" That was that, as far as Miller was concerned because it appeared that there was not much she felt she could do and she realized that tears were rolling down her cheeks; most unprofessional and most unpremeditated, but something wondrous then happened. Ionesco asked Miller if he could speak in French and it all suddenly started; she recorded a touching and wonderful interview that lasted an hour, and the recording is one of her most precious possessions from the journalistic period of her career. Unexpectedly, she was also able to put the interview she had recorded for *The Sunday Times* to good use and have it published in dialogue format (question and answer) in an equally prestigious publication, the art magazine *Artforum,* which was edited by maverick editor Ingrid Sischy (who died tragically in 2015 aged 63) and she chose a fabulous title for Miller's interview: "Excuse Me Madame but It Seems to Me Unless I'm Mistaken That I've Met You Somewhere Before: A Conversation with Eugène Ionesco by Sanda Miller" (*Artforum* March 1987 pp. 94-98).

Peter McNeil "attempts" to interview Manolo Blahnik.

In mid-2007 Anja Cronberg, the indefatigable editor of *ACNE Paper* Sweden, asked McNeil to interview the famous shoe designer Manolo Blahnik. This seemed too much of an opportunity to turn down, as McNeil had recently edited a book with economic historian Giorgio Riello on the history of shoes, and Blahnik had graciously provided an endorsement (which had really came from the PR department—as it is so often the case). Apart from flying from Australia to interview Blahnik, no mean feat, McNeil knew what to expect of Blahnik's famous speaking style, which is an over the top staccato of exclamations and pronouncements, moving between past and present and referring to many famous figures from the past, from various countesses to Cecil Beaton and Lady Diana Cooper, whom he had met in his youth. The charming PR person set up a meeting at Blue Bird Members Club, Beaufort St, London, where Blahnik was relaxed, and the interview began. McNeil was aware from the very beginning that Blahnik tended to repeat himself: McNeil had researched all the press and magazine articles that he could find beforehand and many of them contained the same *bon mots*, witticisms, and other observations. As anyone can see in the various documentaries made about fashion and style in which Blahnik appears, he is also a person of great presence and elegance, tall and refined, who has the air of an agitated bird, barely listening to the questions posed to him before darting off in another direction. McNeil decided that the best angle would be to use his own knowledge and respect for fashion figures from the past, and after some small talk about the success of the shoe business, went in at that direction. He also tried to disarm Blahnik through the use of charm:

Blahnik: Professor McNeil, so young, and I loved your book!

McNeil:

Thank you very much; I won't be seeing 40 again. Mr Blahnik, you have been called the "Proust of Shoes." But your early shoes did not play on old-fashioned ideals of inter-war elegance.

Blahnik:

I don't like madeleines. I hate it. Oh well. I don't like that label. I've never liked rooms full of cork, I can't stand being confined in one place and I can't stand housekeepers, so Céleste, it was not for me at all. This is just one of the things they call you. Once at a dinner Calvin Klein said to me, "My Darling Moz-art of the shoes"—[indicates with a gesture that he means the composer—slight aside]. I laugh about everything.

McNeil:

Let's play with this idea of elegance. Is it fixed? Some American fashion designers that I have talked to have a very rigid notion of elegance.

Blahnik:

Like what—Babe Paley—uhh—kind of boring.... Babe Paley was a wonderful woman but Millicent Rogers was much more spunky than Babe Paley was. Millicent Rogers was a wonderful designer, she did incredible affairs and incredible things and amazing designs wearing dresses designed by her. She went to Austria and New Mexico, did amazing things with huge jewels on her cravats. Mrs Paley was [gestures grandly] one of those things that has gone now forever, that one. They have all gone, including the modern versions like Mrs Buckley, Mrs Kempner, who have gone now, they've all gone. Babe Paley was one of those things that we don't have ever more. New York has gone, Mrs de la Renta is left, I adore her, but New York is gone. Anyway I've seen some awful pumps there in the 70s with soles by Du Pont. Can you imagine?

Blahnik had responded, and began to open up a bit. So McNeil obtained something fresh and new about Blahnik, which did not simply repeat what others had said, and had to distill a great deal of words where there was never a conclusion to the sentence, into prose that made sense. At the same time he wished to capture the charming spirit of this creative genius, and be respectful without sycophantic. He knew that Blahnik was an aesthete, but sometimes the answers were unexpected:

McNeil: *Do you love looking at the art or act of walking?*

Blahnik: Statues. Well let's talk about statues! I am interested in statues, the interpretation of someone like Praxiteles. *Voilà!* Anybody!—I love it! As a boy I went to the Prado, I couldn't care about the paintings, always I looked at the statues. For instance, Canova; Pauline Borghese; and the warriors, so sensual, that they found in the water, I could die, I love feet. I don't care about any part of the body—I'm doing this [designing shoes] because it's all I care about—apart from maybe the eyes.

This is a hard feat to achieve with many fashion designers, who tend to repeat the same thing—as do many artists and other creative individuals—and the only way around this is to have done the research before arriving at the interview, as it will be impossible to redirect the conversation otherwise.

How to interview?

Adams and Hicks provide detailed practical advice about interviewing, starting with preparation, the use of equipment, the ideal type of questions, all of which are based on their extensive practice, which ultimately amounts to learning on a trial-and-error basis (their own). Whether such a system can be generalized to become an accepted system of teaching journalism remains a matter of debate, but there is no doubt that sharing has many benefits, even if the shared experience as something very personal cannot become a trusted system of "teaching" journalism. Nevertheless, there are some well-established general rules in journalism such as the six key questions, referenced by Adams and Hicks as well as Randall, which suggest that they can be regarded as a modest theoretical foundation for teaching journalist skills.

The bulk of their advice is common sense and practical assistance, which provides help, but most importantly, encouragement for the journalist, because it would be too frightening to find yourself facing an interviewee without having a prepared strategy. In the event that prepared strategy is thrown out the window because you are facing such an unexpected situation, as Miller did when she interviewed the great playwright Eugène Ionesco, the journalist needs to have the ability to think on their feet, and fast too, because no textbook or advice can prepare anybody for the unexpected, with the difference that an experienced journalist is always prepared. But for the beginner this can be a matter of succeeding or failing—it is as simple as this!

The starting point must always be rigorous preparation (plan, research, be punctual), then move on to the interview itself (listen, empathize) they consider to be key principles, which "underpin the successful interviews" (Adams and Hicks, 2009: 12–13). But a good interview does not only depend on preparation and good questions, for they give advice on issues such as "arriving on time," shaking hands, eye contact, even where to sit, which as bizarre as it may appear is important because as part of the strategy of good interviewing practice:

> If this is your first interview, sit where indicated. Later, with growing experience and confidence, you can be more choosey—because where you sit matters. Accepted wisdom is that sitting directly opposite your interviewee is a mistake. It's confrontational, the chess or "war" position. Sitting too far away is a mistake, too, as is sitting side by side on the

sofa ... There's general agreement that sitting at about right-angles (90 degrees) works best, being neither confrontational nor cosy. (Adams and Hicks, 2009: 35)

Miller was able to confirm this piece of advice from her personal experience before reading Adams and Hicks's book, which only goes to show that even if journalism does not benefit from an accepted theoretical framework an equally important code of practice disseminated orally is beginning to make its way into books as this example demonstrates.

Miller started to work for BBC (Radio 3) as a researcher and compiler for documentaries for famed producer Piers Plowright and they collaborated between 1984 and 1997. Their last program (just before his retirement) was entitled "What are they looking at?" and was based on Jan van Eyck's masterpiece in the National Gallery (London) entitled "The Arnolfini Wedding" (1434); the program received the "Sony Award" (bronze) for 1997. Miller's job (and yes journalism is work) was to interview the people that were selected for documentaries, and between 1984 and 1998 Miller researched and compiled nine 45-minute such art documentaries for which she received training regarding interviewing techniques from the BBC. One of the most important things was "where to sit," which was considered as a useful strategy for radio interviews which could take place anywhere, not just in the studios of the BBC at Broadcasting House. What she learnt confirms what Adams and Hicks wrote, namely that the best strategy would be to sit at an angle of 90 degrees, which, Miller's teacher joked, could even enable one "to play footsy with the interviewee."

Feet aside, in terms of preparing the questions for an interview, the most important issue is research, because if the interviewer is perceived not to be totally in control of the subject matter, that would be not only embarrassing but unprofessional.

In chapter IV (pp. 39–70) of their book Adams and Hicks offer advice on interviewing whereby "interviewers need to master the non-questioning skills of eliciting information and quotes. These are: listen and encourage, make statements requiring confirmation/denial and finally summarise and move on" (Adams and Hicks, 2001: 39).

To return to Miller's interview with Eugène Ionesco, the one thing she did know were Ionesco's plays as well as the post-World War II period of existentialist despair which informed them, because what Ionesco shared was not about his comedic dialogue style but the uselessness of language as a tool of human communication, which ultimately breaks down:

As time has passed, the language of my plays has deteriorated more and more—in my last one, *Voyages chez les morts* (Journeys among the dead), the last-act monologue of the main character is composed of assonances, of made-up words, disarticulated utterances. It is no

more than a sort of crying. Facing the realization of the hopelessness
of communication, the deterioration of language, the degradation of
all human relationships. I could do only one thing: make my language
more and more denunciatory, in fact make it into an antilanguage, a false
language. (Artforum, 1987: 97)

Miller used her interview in two ways: the first commissioned written
for a newspaper took the shape of a profile, introduced as "a report"
complemented by a wonderful photograph of Ionesco by Sally Soames.
Miller made good use of Ionesco's answers, such as his pessimistic view
regarding language as an inadequate means of communication given in the
above quote and she was able to follow it with her own comments regarding
Ionesco's beginnings:

Language has always been at the centre of Ionesco's work. He began to
write plays as a consequence of teaching himself English with the Assimil
conversation manual; when his double-bill of "The Bald Prima Donna"
and "The Lesson" which used some of the manual's stilted dialogue,
opened in 1952 at the Théâtre de la Huchette, he was furiously attacked
as the pioneer of the Theatre of the Absurd. Now he is a grand old man of
drama, a member of the Académie Française and rather out of sympathy
with contemporary theatre (Sanda Miller: *The Sunday Times*, November
30, 1986, p. 51)

What was particularly enjoyable was that she was able to structure the
article by following a classical format (also used by Jo Ellisson in her
profile of Tom Ford for the *FT*) by starting with a description of Ionesco,
something that an interview published in dialogue form does not allow,
then moving on to his *oeuvre* and the motivation behind his writing, as well
as his views on politics which played an important part in his career as he
disliked *le théâtre engagé,* and in particular the Marxist slant displayed in
Bertolt Brecht's plays.

This is how Ionesco was introduced to the readers:

Frail, impeccably dressed, the Romanian-born Ionesco seems protected
from the troubles of the world by the surroundings of his elegant
apartment on Boulevard Montparnasse, almost directly above the
Coupole brasserie—but it is an impression quickly dispelled by the
solemnity of his statements. His very large, very expressive eyes shine
as he speaks (Sanda Miller: *The Sunday Times*, November 30, 1986, p.
51).

For *Artforum*, Miller published her entire interview question and answer,
beautifully edited by the late Sischy, who wrote an introduction about
how Miller came about to interview Ionesco and instructions as to how to

"recite" the interview—clearly an imaginary situation in keeping with the theatre of the absurd—a contribution Miller treasures:

> One day last summer, years after I had first seen his work, I woke up with him on my mind, as one wakes up having dreamed abut people, not remembering the dream but with a sense of their presence. It seemed important to talk to Ionesco and the following interview is the result (Sanda Miller).
> *(The dialogue which follows must be spoken in voices that are drawling, monotonous, a little singsong, without nuances)*
> (Sanda Miller, 1987:92)

Adams and Hicks offer sensible and useful advice about interviewing techniques in chapter IV of their book which consists not only in the way questions should ideally be framed but also practical advice for the interviewers such as eye contact, body language, friendliness, etc., and Miller was pleased that a lot of what she learnt from personal experience on the basis of trial and error rather than reading specialist books on journalism made her reach similar conclusions. In the case of Ionesco, she was also lucky that once he started to speak she needed to do little else but listen and listen because what he had to say was so moving that as to render her speechless. Below is one of the many wonderful replies which refers to Martin Esslin's invention of the label "the theatre of the absurd" Ionesco did not condone but neither did he fully reject it:

> When it was said that my generation of authors were authors of the absurd, we accepted the label because of the recognition that came with it. But more generally I accepted "the absurd" as a label because I told myself that after all Martin Esslin, who wrote the book *The Theatre of the Absurd* had a point; the world is absurd, or is rendered absurd by man. The idea of the absurd has existed for a long time, and its real father is Shakespeare, who had Macbeth say: "Life's but a walking shadow, a poor player/ That struts and frets his hour upon the stage/ And then is heard no more; it is a tale/Told by an idiot, full of sound and fury,/ Signifying nothing." This is why I consider Shakespeare the great ancestor of the theatre of the absurd. (Miller, 1987: 96)

An important piece of advice regarded even as a "rite of passage" for the interviewer, on offer from Adams and Hicks, was that in planning an interview, journalists must familiarize themselves with news:

> you must learn to sniff out news. The approach is quite simple: jump right in at the deep end. It's not easy for beginners. In fact it can be downright difficult and embarrassing, but it happens to the best, and once you're out and on the other side, you're on your way. (Adams and Hicks, 2009: 9)

The example they offer is none other than the wonderful Andrew Marr,[1] who started his journalistic career as trainee reporter on a local paper, reminiscing about it:

> We were sent off to local villages and outlying suburbs ... and told not to come back until we had half a dozen publishable stories ... That meant slowly scrubbing away any natural shyness, banging on vicars' doors, stopping shopkeepers and pleading with councillors for anything— anything. Stray dog? Upset at the Guild? Older villager? (Adams and Hicks, 2009: 9)

From stray dogs to interviewing heads of state, presidents, and practically the most important men on this earth, it is only one of the many examples of a glamorous trajectory, but then, not every journalist is Andrew Marr either. Yet for the majority who do wish to embark on the exciting and demanding career of being a journalist, this is a career which can offer both professional success and personal satisfaction.

The review

Is there such a thing as a fashion review? Unexpected perhaps, this question is nevertheless legitimate for one important reason: reviewing is the work of the critic and the critic generally writes about art. Granted that to even attempt to provide a logical definition, in the sense of establishing necessary and sufficient conditions for something to be thus defined, is an impossible task. The reason? The reason is to do with the way we define art which started to change—even before Marcel Duchamp unleashed his "ready-mades" onto the art world in 1913 declaring them art (because I Marcel Duchamp say so!)—with the arrival of photography and film; but that was only the beginning, for we can confidently add fashion to the list. Today, it is generally accepted that some photography and films are art, although in the majority of cases we still speak of design, craft, trade, business, etc., because nobody in their right mind would call all commercial photography or blockbuster films art, nor should they. The argument can be extended to fashion, given that although in some instances fashion can be considered art, we are in fact dealing with a vast commercial enterprise.

We find ample examples of photography and film reviews in the press but we are yet to find a fashion review, although major fashion exhibitions held at the foremost museums (as well as festivals such as Hyères) in the world are now being reviewed, not only in specialized magazines, but

---

[1]Andrew William Stevenson Marr (born 1959) is a distinguished journalist and television presenter who was editor of *The Independent and* BBC News and at present hosts the very successful TV program *The Andrew Marr Show* (launched in 2005) every Sunday morning on BBC One.

also in the national press. This however is not the case with the fashion show. The fashion show is not generally **reviewed**; the fashion show is **reported**. It is often the only fashion-related component of an evening news broadcast or splash page of an online newspaper. Nor is this a mere matter of semantics as we intend to prove, because we are dealing with two distinct activities that require a type of expertise which differs from that of the critic.

Before we choose our examples we would like to reference again Caroline Evans's *Fashion at the Edge* (2003), whose subtitle "Spectacle, Modernity and Deathliness" reflects the main areas of discussion with the section on "Spectacle" (pp. 65–86) dedicated to the fashion show. Her focus is on three of the most creative fashion designers of the 1990s—John Galliano, Alexander McQueen, and Hussein Chalayan, among others—and to her list she adds the name of Martin Margiela, whose fashion shows can arguably be regarded more as art installations and performances whereby instead of choosing the glamor of the fashion show, Margiela held his in derelict urban spaces such as "car parks, disused metro stations, warehouses and wasteland" (Evans, 2003: 80).

But what is the real function of the fashion show, for whichever way we look at it, a fashion show is neither an art installation, nor a performance, nor any other form of art; a fashion show (unless otherwise framed) is just a fashion show plain and simple. For this reason we must not forget its main function: advertising with a view to selling a new collection (we concede there are parades staged particularly as a part of research investigations within the art and design school setting, but these are research or practice-based investigations and not commercial affairs).

'Fashion Journalism' especially in terms of practical advice about how to report a fashion show. Bradford starts by referencing "the good old times," when Grace Coddington was a fashion reporter for *US Vogue*, which not only makes for nostalgic reading but reveals how the practice of fashion reporting has changed (but not—according to Coddington—for the better, because she found the current approach less than inspirational). In fact, at the time when her autobiographical book *A Memoir* was published in 2012, she had made up her mind about the brave new world of fashion reporting: "I can't stand it" (Coddington (2012) in Bradford, 2015: 127).

But in what sense did the style of fashion reporting change? What Coddington was deploring was the passing of the sincerity and simplicity of the fashion show and its public alike. Gone were the times when editors sat in deep sofas or gilt chairs and "stately models came on holding cards with the number of their outfit on," and this was more or less it: "there was no music, no scenario, and no drama to distract you from examining the clothes. It was one hundred percent about the clothes" (Bradford, 2015).

From the young woman carrying a card with a number on it to the spectacular events costing millions of pounds on offer from the likes of Lagerfeld, there is indeed a world of difference. The conclusion that emerges is that for many the fashion show really has to be dedicated to clothes and not pretend to be something else.

Bradford provides also useful advice on writing about fashion shows and how they continue to be regularly reported by the press, including

> quality newspapers like *The Times, Independent, Daily Telegraph* and *Guardian*, and on the websites of glossies like *Vogue, Grazia* and *Elle*. Tabloid newspapers and weekly magazines are more likely to cover them from the point of view of which celebrities show up in the front row, rather than send a reporter out to review them. The Chanel autumn-winter 2013 show, for instance, got widespread coverage when not only Rihanna but film start Kristen Stewart turned up. (Bradford, 2015: 128–9)

We selected two examples on the topics of parades, both from the national press: the first is an extended report by Suzy Menkes on the Paris Fashion Show (Friday September 28) in the *Global Edition of the New York Times* 2012 entitled "Generation Genius" (pp. 9–12). Its very title reflects Menkes's admiration for the quality of the collections on display, and she starts by showering prize on Nicolas Ghesquière's latest collection for Balenciaga:

> Mr. Ghesquière's Balenciaga has been 15 years in the making. But he has never offered such a confident vision. He took the rigor of the founder; the steely geometry of his cut—swirling, Spanish shapes—and mixed all that with a 21st century freedom of flesh. "It's my most sensual collection; I wanted to show more skin and to express the duality between movement and mobility, between Cubism and dance," the designer said.

But that one collection was given pride of place was Dior, Menkes called: "a triumph of 21st century modernism" and that triumph was the creation of Raf Simons:

> In the designer's hands, rigid lines melted into rounded shapes, tailored coats broken out into pleats and luminous fabrics reflected, literally and metaphorically, a change of mood. "I am rethinking the idea of minimalism to be sensual and sexual, fun and free," Mr. Simons said. "I looked back to Mr. Dior's period after the war and then at the whole idea in the '60s and '70s of psychological and sexual freedom and liberation."

Menkes also referred to Alber Elbaz, the Israeli designer working for Lanvin, with whom she concluded her sparkling report:

> And Mr. Elbaz always adds a touch of nonchalant wit about being a woman as in a handbag in the shape of a perfume bottle: a goddess for the 21st century.

For our second example we turn to a curiously "populist" approach we found in *The Times*. We selected a report from the "Met Gala" (*The Times*, May 4, 2016 pp. 4–5) by Harriet Walker entitled "Body armour and buttocks: what happened when style went sci-fi," whose subtitle was "Hairdos like phone masts, tin foil frocks—it must be the Met Gala." It becomes immediately obvious that the frivolous content, fluffy style of reporting, as well as the angle of approach are to do with money and more money and how much tickets cost (we are looking at something like £20,000 at least for a ticket). We would call this piece a reportage, whose aims and objectives were to convey how the great and the good celebrate a fashion event, in this instance the Metropolitan Museum of Art's latest exhibition: *Manus x Machina: Fashion in the Age of Technology*. No doubt it was a worthwhile and also very popular exhibition with the cognoscenti, but this newspaper review is not about the merits or otherwise of the latest offering on fashion from a world-class museum but rather the circus of the "Met Gala":

Cindy Crawford and Jourdan Dunn sparkled in their full-length, silver-tiled Balmain gowns, but in hers Kim Kardashian looked more like a shish kebab made of disco balls. It was reminiscent of a suit of Henry VIII's armour I once saw in a museum. Apparently he had to be winched on to his horse while wearing it—look out for something similar on her reality show.

Bradford gives useful advice about fashion reporting that parallels the practical advice on offer when preparing for an interview, and she starts with the all-important issue of the specialized vocabulary needed in fashion reporting:

Take a look at the references any catwalk report on, say, *Style.com* and you'll see the wealth knowledge at the fingertips of the writers. A Tim Blanks review of an Alexander McQueen show, for instance, has the cultural references of Madame Grès (early twentieth-century French couturier), Fortuny (early twentieth-century Spanish designer), Gaudi (Spanish architect), Gaia (Ancient Greek goddess) and the trademarks of earlier McQueen shows. It refers to fabrics like matelassé jacquard, silk chiffon, lace and organza, embellishments like appliqué, pleating and ruffles, and cuts like trapeze and the Empire line. (Bradford, 2015: 132)

After useful practical advice about how to gain access to such shows by acquiring accreditation from the official organization, for example, British Fashion Council in London to attend the show, she adds a humorous comment regarding the arcane system of seating. In terms of reporting, Bradford offers advice about "What you're looking for in a show" and "How to write up a catwalk report," and at this point we wish to point out that as with all our own examples both in print and fashion journalism, the advice that authors have on offer is their own personal experience, where the common denominator is knowledge and clarity of expression. Thus, in the case of the former, Bradford lists the following key headings to look for: "the designer's inspiration," "context," "a key look or theme," "production" (e.g., if the show is particularly lavish then that should become "the angle of the piece," and indeed with an example such as that of Karl Lagerfeld importing an iceberg from Sweden for the Chanel autumn-winter show of 2010, the Swedish iceberg had to take center stage). More lighthearted approaches can also be adopted, such as "Celebrity" (who sits in the front row, Victoria Beckham or Joe Bloggs), but we feel that the heading "Verdict" comes closest to the job of the critic:

> If a collection was scintillatingly brilliant, or especially awful, that can form the angle of the piece. Because a bad review is far less common that a good one, a negative verdict is particularly newsworthy. Jess Cartner-Morley started her review of Tom Ford's spring-summer 2012 show like this "I'm going to come straight out with it. Deep breath: I didn't think Tom Ford's show as all that. Not that it was awful, by any means, but despite the beautiful tailoring and immaculate execution, it fell a little flat. It felt too self-referential". (Cartner-Morley in Bradford, 2015: 140)

We have to smile at this elegant pussy-footing, for Ms. Cartner-Morley is not even remotely critical of the grand Tom Ford, how could she, for had she presumed to behave otherwise, she would lose her job in a minute. In this respect the art world is more objective in the sense that critics do say it as it is, and in the United Kingdom we had an excellent example in the late Brian Sewell (1931–2015), who was the art critic of the *Evening Standard* from 1984 to his death. For years Sewell spat venom on so many artists that this had the unexpected outcome that instead of fearing his ire, artists started to fear that a positive review would spell disaster and lower their standing in the art world. Sewell was threatened, thrown out from various galleries—one famous example being the all-powerful Anthony d'Offay Gallery (1965–2001), which was showing such international luminaries as Andy Warhol and Joseph Beuys. Yet Sewell's position as critic writing for the *Evening Standard* was secure, and he kept it until his death in 2015.[2]

Indeed, how critical can the fashion critic be? This is the moot question that Bradford deals with next, and it seems that even if the critic tries to be critical it will not cut much water in the world of fashion:

> Magazines cannot be critical of advertisers in print ... That, together with publication dates, means that their catwalk coverage is more likely to

---

[2]On Sewell's background in Art History and also the auction rooms, see his autobiography *Outsider: Always Almost: Never Quite, An Autobiography*, London: Quartet Books, 2011.

be of the round-up variety (in weeklies) trend reports (in weeklies and monthlies) and shoots. If a collection is judged to be poor, it will simply get fewer mentions, or none at all. As Elizabeth Walker, former executive fashion editor at *Maire Claire* says: "Magazines comment by omission. If one show is dreadful, you might use one picture because they did show, but that's all." (Bradford, 2015: 141)

But there is help at hand from newspapers, which are not so dependent on advertising, and in this respect some of the finest fashion writers, including Hilary Alexander, Cathy Horyn, and Suzy Menkes, all had the courage to be critical, although they too had to pay a price, not dissimilar to that of Brian Sewell. Thus, "Suzy Menkes was banned from all LVMH shows on a single day in October 2001 after a critical review of Dior." It was the British fashion critic Colin McDowell, who, together with Cathy Horyn (both writing for the *New York Times*), were banned by Armani because of their reviews of the collection:

Colin McDowell responded by writing ferociously about the sensitivity of fashion brands and the effect it has on critical journalism. In a column for the *Business of Fashion*, he wrote that there were fewer than half a dozen writers who were prepared to voice an opinion: "And that's because the sanctions for speaking the truth are severe, because if they are not, the entire self-congratulatory smoke and mirrors, candy floss edifice of fashion could collapse into an unedifying goo," he added. (Bradford, 2015: 142)

Finally, to the question "Do we still need the shows?" It seems that whether we need them or not, they are out there for all of us to see. But even in this respect we notice a radical change whereby these exclusive events reserved for the great and the good have altered to become popular shows good enough for Guy Debord's book *The Society of Spectacle* (1967), or rather its epigons, and that change has come from the Internet:

By 2010, the Internet enabled London Fashion Week to start live-streaming shows online. Several years later, most shows were shown live on the likes of Facebook, YouTube, magazine websites and the brands' own sites. From 2011, the website NOWFASHION (wwwnowfashion. com) also posted photographs from runway shows and presentations almost in real time. (Bradford, 2015: 143)

Magazines appear to still contain elements of resistance to the "democratization" of opinion; consider the scandal of 2016 in which important editors at Vogue "declared war" on and suggested that the bloggers were ignorant hangers-on "in borrowed clothes" (https://www. theguardian.com/media/2016/sep/29/vogue-editors-declare-war-fashion-bloggers accessed November 24, 2016). But the fashion industry is a true survivor, for they were the first to acknowledge, even welcome, the new mode of presenting fashion to the world:

> Those in fashion also argue that the shows are an important coming-together of the industry, where everyone mingles, networks and learns where their place is. "It's a really important way of keeping the industry together" says *Grazia*'s Hannah Almassi. (Bradford, 2015: 144)

Blogging is a cultural phenomenon that demands its own investigation separate from ours. Many bloggers are not journalists, and whether they are producing journalism or opinion needs to be analyzed and debated. Many instagrammers state "I am not a blogger" on their sites. The fact that distinctions such as these have emerged is fascinating in itself as it seems to suggest that they do not wish to be tainted with a commercial association. But most bloggers are also not commercial or being "sponsored" as the euphemism goes (this language will need to be explained to future generations). Can we not conclude then, thinking back to the debates that once raged about exposing the general public to Salon art and culture in its many other manifestations, from theatre to ballet and cinema, that this is very much a case of "plus ça change plus c'est la même chose"?

Conclusion

Journalism emerged as a means of communication long before the news-books (*corantos*)—the first of which is dated 1513. One such example of proto-news is the "pasquinade," defined by *Collins English Dictionary* as "an abusive lampoon or satire posted in a public place." The name "pasquinade" is derived from an ancient Roman statue disinterred in Rome in 1501 that was affectionately nicknamed "Pasquino." Pasquino became the equivalent of "Private Eye" (a best-selling UK current-affairs newspaper), because the aspiring satirical journalists who pioneered this genre would post their verses on the statue for all to read and ridicule. No wonder that one of the first such writers was the fearless Pietro Aretino, nicknamed "the scourge of princes," discussed in this book in Chapter 2, because nobody escaped his biting satire. If he felt like lampooning a political personality, a famous writer, painter, sculptor, or musician, he would pour his venom on his victim, and what better example than his astonishingly nasty rant against the divine Michelangelo!

Despite the derivation of news in very old practices connected to public notes and broadsheets (an English term for a one pager posted up in the street or on a tree) we can confidently regard *The Times* as the first newspaper in the modern sense of the word. First published in 1785 as "The Daily Universal Register" it took its current name in 1788. Nicknamed "the thunderer," the newspaper acquired the reputation of bastion of justice and "fair play"! Sadly, in this instance we can truthfully lament: "oh, how times have changed" (in Cicero's immortal words: "O tempora, o mores!" [Oh the times! Oh the customs!]), when in 1981, "the thunderer" was taken over by Rupert Murdoch's *News International* which prompted its editor of fourteen years, William Rees-Mogg, to resign.[1] The mighty "thunderer" has become today a rather meek moaner and perhaps *The Times* gave us a taste

---

[1]He was promptly replaced by Harold Evans, chosen by Murdoch himself.

of what was to come in terms of emasculating the freedom of information that the press once jealously guarded as their most precious privilege.

But change was a-foot yet again, because in the age of the Internet and fast communication we no longer rely on either broadsheets or tabloids for news, gossip, art reviews, fashion reports, the weather forecast, or indeed the all important sport. We now have an array of little devices to which we are all hooked (note the early morning commuters who instead of literally hiding behind the protective opened broadsheets [that format has barely survived but for a few examples] which totally covered their faces and half their bodies); instead, the commuters are now either wired to their mobile, or read their tablets on which they may (or may not) have downloaded articles from their favored newspaper. The printed word is still among us but in a modified format, for many cities now have newspapers which are distributed for free. Thus, in London we have "Metro," a free sheet tabloid published by DMG Media (part of Daily Mail and General Trust) filled mostly with the latest shenanigans of the "celebs" which saturate its unpleasantly designed pages while news and important reports are kept to a minimum. It was founded in 1999 as the free newspaper you could collect from stands on your way to work, at that date a novelty, and when it was launched it was impressive. A process of deterioration started gradually to erode the quality of its content, and now it is a rather miserable "rag" (from "rag paper") whose contents seem to be vaguely flicked over by most readers, but its power is insidious. This is because many commuters pick it up for a few minutes instead of buying a quality newspaper. For that reason "Metro" can be arguably seen as one of the many factors why print journalism is in decline, although we firmly believe that this is only a historical moment and the proverbial pendulum will swing back to quality writing at some point in the future.

In the afternoon we have *The Evening Standard* in London, a much better proposition whose origins go back 180 years to 1827, when it was founded as *The Standard* by barrister Stanley Lees Giffard. It was published as *The Evening Standard* until 2009 when it became *The London Evening Standard* mainly owned by charismatic Evgeny Lebedev (about 63 percent), while the rest belongs to the *Daily Mail* and *General Trust*.

We noticed an interesting change in the system of communication whereby the ever increasing size of the broadsheets, which began (some still do) to approximate the size of a double-decker London bus, have lost their interest (and justifiably too, as the readership was mostly pumped with trivia). They have been replaced with a bullet-point system called Google (an electronic British Library, Library of Congress, or Bibliothèque Nationale contained in a mobile) that feeds us all the information, no matter how obscure, in dot-point format. This is not all bad, because all we need is this essential information (its contents greatly exceed that of an Encyclopedia) on which we can expand by using "traditional" research methods that tertiary training provides us.

As we arrived at the final moments of creating this book, the world witnessed the sudden emergence of the expressions "fake news," "alternative facts," and "post truth"—the first coined by the new American President Donald Trump to attack venerable news organizations, including the New York Times, NCN News, ABC, CBS and CNN; "alternative facts" coined by Trump's Counselor Kellyanne Conway in January 2017 to suggest some facts were better than others, and the latter used to suggest that the truth is no longer discernible. As others have remarked, this is also "back to the future" (our expression): Richard Nixon said in the 1960s: "The Press is the enemy … The establishment is the enemy, the professors are the enemy" (*USA Today*, http://www.usatoday.com/story/news/politics/onpolitics/2017/02/17/trump-news-media-enemy-american-people/98065338/ accessed 18 February 2017). There is a grim irony in much of this noted by others: that some of the effects of post-modernism and post-structuralism—at first influential only in the Academy—approaches that questioned grand narratives, "truth" as a white, western construction and the like, have now been co-opted by the Right Wing of politics to suggest that the line between reality and illusion is no more (Jean Baudrillard had in fact been correct). We know all this because in the age of relativism, truth itself ceased to be absolute and post-modernism with its "incredulity" toward meta-narratives is best placed to confirm its relevance to our times. To this we would add that Pontus Pilate, too, knew this when he famously asked "What is Truth!," but did not stay for an answer. The president is already infamous for becoming the first such leader in history to communicate policy formation mainly via social media platforms of twitter and tweets, bypassing the norms of communication expected of his office.

In the age of technology when communication is faster than ever via the Internet, information at our fingertips via Google and visual information surrounds us to the point of saturation on billboards, on posters, on tables, on the little screens of our mobiles, few of us have time to commune for several hours a day with the elegant subtleties of good quality journalism (it takes several hours to read a quality newspaper cover to cover). But we can admire also how the style of communication has gone full circle: by comparing these bullet-pointed bits of information with the *pasquinades*. There is no doubt that Pietro Aretino's scatological sense of humor has its contemporary equivalents; nor do we have to search for too long to find them. We can indeed say how things have changed and not necessarily for the worse, but we can also say that in true dialectical fashion we have today returned to the system of communication pioneered by the mischievous bulletin posters: short, sharp, and not necessarily sweet!

BIBLIOGRAPHY AND FURTHER READING

Adams, S. and W. Hicks (2009), *Interviewing for Journalists*, London and New York: Routledge.

Appleby, J. et al., eds. (1996), *Knowledge and Postmodernism in Historical Perspective*, New York: Routledge.

Aretino, P. ([1534] 1971), *The Ragionamenti*: *The Erotic Lives of Nuns, Wives and Courtesans*, London: Panther Books.

Aretino, P. (1976), *Selected Letters*, Harmondsworth and New York: Penguin.

Barber, L., ed. (2015), *Lunch with the FT* (52 Classic Interviews), Portfolio Penguin.

Barnard, M., ed. (2007), *Fashion Theory: A Reader*, Routeldge.

Barry, P. (2001), *Beginning Theory*: *An Introduction to Literary and Cultural Theory*, Manchester: Manchester University Press.

Barthes, R. ([1967] 1990), *The Fashion System*, Berkeley: University of California Press.

Bartlett Djurdja, Shaun Cole, and Agnes Rocamora (eds.): Fashion Media (Past and Present, Bloomsbury, 2013.

Baudelaire, C. (1972), *Selected Writings on Art and Artists*, Harmondsworth: Penguin Books.

Beardsley, M. C. (1966), *Aesthetics from Classical Greece to the Present: A Short History*, New York: The Macmillan Company.

Berg, M. and Helen Clifford (2007), "Selling Consumption in the Eighteenth Century: Advertising and the Trade Card in Britain and France," *Cultural and Social History*, 4(2): 145–170.

Berry, D. (2012), *Journalism: Ethics and Society*, Farnham and Burlington: Ashgate Publishing.

Berry, D. and J. Theobald, eds. (2006), *Radical Mass Media Criticism (A Cultural Genealogy)*, Montreal and New York: Black Rose Books.

Bissonette, A. (2015), "*Dessiné d'après nature*: Renditions from Life in the *Journal des Dames et des Modes* 1798–1799," *Journal for Eighteenth-Century Studies*, 38(2): 213–237.

Boehn, M. von. ([1929] 1972), *Dolls*, New York: Dover. Republication of the one-vol., trans. J. Nicoll, *Dolls and Puppets*, n.d. first published in 2 vols. in German.

Borsay, Peter (1989), *The English Urban Renaissance. Culture and Society in the Provincial Town 1660–1770*. Oxford: Oxford University Press.

Bottéro, J. (2004), *The Oldest Cuisine in the World. Cooking in Mesopotamia*, trans. T. Lavender Fagan (2002), Chicago and London: Chicago University Press.

Boucher, F. (1997), *A History of Costume in the West*, Thames and Hudson. Collins English Dictionary (2005), Collins (seventh edition).

Bradford, J. (2015), *Fashion Journalism*, Abington: Routledge.

Branston, G. and R. Stafford (1998), *The Media Student's Book*, New York: Routledge.

Breward, C. (1994), "Femininity and Consumption: The Problem of the Late Nineteenth-Century Fashion Journal," *Journal of Design History*, 7(2): 71–89.

Brewer, J. (1997), *The Pleasure of the Imagination: English Culture in the Eighteenth Century*, New York: Farrar, Straus & Giroux.

Briggs, A. (1994), *A Social History of England*, London: Weidenfeld and Nicholson.

Burke, E. (1990), *A Philosophical Enquiry into the Origin of Our Ideas of the Sublime and Beautiful*, New York: Oxford University Press.

Butler, C. ([2004] 2009), *Pleasure and the Arts. Enjoying Literature, Painting and Music*, Oxford: Oxford University Press.

Carter, M. (2006), *Fashion Classics: From Carlyle to Barthes*, London: Berg.

Censer, Jack R. (1994), *The French Press in the Age of Enlightenment*, London and New York: Routledge.

Chisick, Harvey (1991). "Introduction," in Harvey Chisick with Ilana Zinger and Ouzi Elyada (ed.), *The Press in the French Revolution*, Oxford: University of Oxford and The Voltaire Foundation.

Croizat, Y. C. (2007), "'Living Dolls': François I Dresses His Women," *Renaissance Quarterly*, 60(1): 94–130.

Davies, M. (1997), *Europe: A History*, New York: Pimlico.

Debord, G. (1995), *The Society of the Spectacle*, New York: Zone Books.

de Certeau, M. (1984), *The Practice of Everyday Life I*, trans. S. F. Rendall California: University of California Press.

de la Motte Fouqué, C. (1987), *Geschichte der Moden, 1785–1829*, Berlin: Union Verlag.

D. Jones: (2012) 'The Donatella Interview', Vogue online, 31 May, but as I found this in Bradford, the note should be altered to: Jones in Bradford, 2012: 11).

Downing Peter, Lauren (2017), "'Fashion Plus': Pose and the Plus-Size Body in Vogue, 1986–1988," *Fashion Theory*, 21(2): 175–199.

Eagleton, T. (1992), *The Ideology of the Aesthetic*, Oxford and Cambridge: Blackwell.

Esslin, M. (1983), *An Anatomy of Drama*, Abacus. London.

Evans, M. (2003), *Fashion at the Edge* (Spectacle, Modernity and Deathliness), Yale University Press.

Feagin, S. and P. Maynard (1997), *Aesthetics*, Oxford: Oxford University Press.

Fleming, Juliet (2001), *Graffiti and the Writing Arts of Early Modern England*, Philadelphia: University of Pennsylvania Press.

Fortunato, P. (2009), *Modernist Aesthetics and Consumer Culture in the Writings of Oscar Wilde*, London and New York: Routledge.

Guirand, F. and J. Schmidt, eds. (2006), *Mythes Mythologie: Histoire et dictionnaire*, Larousse. Paris.

Hale, J. (1994), *The Civilization of Europe in the Renaissance*, London: Fontana Press.

Hamlyn, D. W. (1971), *The Theory of Knowledge: Modern Introduction to Philosophy*, London: Macmillan.

Hampsher-Monk, I. (1992), *A History of Modern Political Thought: Major Political Thinkers from Hobbes to Marx*, Oxford and Cambridge: Blackwell.

Harrison, C., P. Wood, and J. Gainger (2000), *Art in Theory 1648–1815* (An Anthology of Changing Ideas), Blackwell, Oxford.

Hartnoll, P. (1985), *The Theatre* (A Concise History), Thames and Hudson, London.

Healy, R. (1982), "Fashion and Textiles Collection," *Art & Australia. Australian National Gallery Special Number*, 20 (1): 98–101.

Hicks, W., S. Adams, H. Gilbert, and T. Holmes (2008), *Writing for Journalists*, London and New York: Routledge.

Holden, Susan (2008), "Kinetic Movement and the Centre Pompidou," in Ursula de Jong and David Beynon (eds), *History in Practice: 25th Annual Conference of the Society of Architectural Historians*, Australia and New Zealand, Geelong, Victoria: published via CD.

Hume, D. (1965), *Of the Standard of Taste and Other Essays*, Indianapolis: The Library of Liberal Arts published by Bobbs-Merrill Company.

Hume, D. (1969), *A Treatise of Human Nature*, Harmondsworth: Penguin Books.

Hume, D. ([1777] 1970), *Enquiries Concerning the Human Understanding and Concerning the Principles of Morals*, Oxford: Oxford University Press.

Jackson, T. and D. Shaw (2006), *The Fashion Handbook*, New York: Routledge.

Johnson, Kim K. P., Susan J. Torntore, and Joanne B. Eicher (eds), *Fashion Foundations. Early Writings on Fashion and Dress*, Oxford and New York: Berg, 2003.

Laver, J. (1969), *A Concise History of Costume*, Thames and Hudson, London.

Marris, P. and S. Thornham (1999), *Media Studies* (A Reader), Edinburgh: Edinburgh University Press.

Marsh, Ian and Gaynor Melville, "Moral Panics and the British Media—A Look at Some Contemporary 'Folk Devils'," *Internet Journal of Criminology*, 2011, http://www.internetjournalofcriminology.com/marsh_melville_moral_panics_and_the_british_media_march_2011.pdf (accessed November 24, 2016).

McDonough, T., ed. (2002), *Guy Debord and the Situationist International; Texts and Documents*, Cambridge, MA: October book, MIT Press.

McKeon, R. (2001), *The Basic Works of Aristotle*, New York.

McNeil, Peter (2007), "Posture: Manolo Blahnik, Shoe Designer" (interview), *ACNE Papers*, "Elegance" issue, 1(5) Autumn 2007: 44–45.

Menchet, M. (2010), *News Reporting and Writing*, Boston: McGraw-Hill Higher Education.

Miller, D. (1987), *Material Culture and Mass Consumption*, Oxford: Basil Blackwell.

Miller, S. (1987), "Excuse Me Madam but It Seems to Me Unless I'm Mistaken that I've Met You Somewhere Before," *Artforum*, March, 92–99.

Miller, S. (1999), "Parody, Pastiche or Purloining? The Uses and Abuses of Artistic Imagery in Media Representations," in D. Berry (ed.), *Ethics and Media Culture* (Practices and Representations), 179–191, Oxford: Focal Press.

Miller, S. (2006), "Armand Mattelart: Historicism and as Media," in D. Berry and J. Theobald (eds), *Radical Mass Media Criticism: A Cultural Genealogy*, Montreal and New York: Black Rose Books.

Miller, S. (2012), "Siegfried Kracauer: Critical Observations on the Discreet Charm of the Metropolis," in D. Berry (ed.), *Revisiting the Frankfurt School: Essays on Culture, Media and Theory*, 7–26, Farnham and Burlington: Ashgate Publishing.

Moeran, Brian (2006), "More than Just a Fashion Magazine," *Current Sociology*, 54(5): 725–744.

Monk, R. and F. Raphael, eds. (2001), *The Great Philosophers: From Socrates to Turing*, London: Phoenix.

Morini, E. (2006), *Storia della moda XVIII-XX secolo*, Skira, Milan.

Motherwell, R. (1972), *Apollinaire on Art, Essays and Reviews 1902–1918 by Guillaume Apollinaire* (The Documents of 20th Century Art), Thames and Hudson, London.

Murphy, Olivia (2013), *Jane Austen the Reader. The Artist as Critic*, New York: Palgrave Macmillan.

Parry, R. (2011), *The Ascent of Media: From Gilgamesh to Google via Gutenberg*, London and Boston: Nicholas Brealey Publishing.

Paul Marris and Sue Thornham: Media Studies: A ReaderEdinburgh University Press, 1996.

Paulicelli, Eugenia (2014), *Writing Fashion in Early Modern Italy. From Sprezzatura to Satire*, Farnham, Surry: Ashgate.

Payne, Michael, ed. (1997), *A Dictionary of Cultural and Critical Theory*, Chichester: Wiley-Blackwell.

Peers, J. (2004), *The Fashion Doll. From Bébé Jumeau to Barbie*, Oxford and New York: Berg.

Peiss, Kathy (2014), *Zoot Suit. The Enigmatic Career of an Extreme Style*, Philadelphia: University of Pennsylvania Press.

Pettegree, A. (2014), *The Invention of News: How the World Came to Know About Itself*, Yale and New Haven: Yale University Press.

Pietsch, Johannes (2013), "On Different Types of Women's Dresses in France in the Louis XVI Period," *Fashion Theory*, 17(4), special suppl.: 397–416.

The Philosopher's Alice: Alice in *Wonderland and Through the Looking-Glass* by Lewis Carroll with illustrations by John Tenniel (Introduction and Notes by Peter Heath), (1974) St. Martin's Press, New York

Potvin, John (2015), "Writing the Dandy Through Art Criticism: Elegance and Civilization in *Monsieur*, 1920–1924," *Fashion Theory*, 20(3): 241–271.

Price, S. (1998), *Media Studies*, London: Longman.

Randall, D. (2011), *The Universal Journalist* (4th edition), London: Pluto Press.

Reponen, J. (2011), "Fashion Criticism Today?," in A. de Witt-Paul and M. Crouch (eds), *Fashion Forward*, Oxford: Interdisciplinary Press ebook.

Ribeiro, A. (1988), *Fashion in the French Revolution*, New York: Holmes and Meier Publishers.

Riello, G. and P. McNeil, eds. (2010), *The Fashion History Reader: Global Perspectives*), Milton Park, Abingdon and New York: Routledge.

Roche, D. (1994), *The Culture of Clothing: Dress and Fashion in the Ancien Régime*, Cambridge: Cambridge University Press.

Rosenthal, M. F. and A. Rosalind Jones (2006), *The Clothing of the Renaissance World: Europe, Asia, Africa, the Americas*, London and New York: Thames and Hudson.

Russell, B. (1976), *The Problems of Philosophy*, Oxford: Oxford University Press.

Ryle, G. ([1949] 1968), *The Concept of Mind*, Harmondsworth: Penguin Books.

Saglio, C. (1913) "Le cinquatenaire de L V P," La vie Parisienne, Samedi, 4 Janvier, p. 3.

Scott, Katie (2004), "Archives and Collections, The Waddesdon Manor Trade Cards: More Than One History." *Journal of Design History,* 17(1): 91–104.

Sewell, Brian (2011), *Outsider: Always Almost: Never Quite, An Autobiography*, London: Quartet Books.

Sheringham, M. (2006), *Everyday Life: Theories and Practices from Surrealism to the Present*, New York: Oxford University Press.

Steele, V. (1996), *Fetish, Fashion, Sex and Power*, Oxford University Press, Oxford.

Stone, Lawrence (1965), *The Crisis of the Aristocracy: 1558–1641*, Oxford: Clarendon Press.

Taylor, L. (2004), *Establishing Dress History*, Manchester: Manchester University Press.

Tétart-Vittu, Françoise, "The Fashion Print: An Ambiguous Object," in Norberg, Kathryn, and Sandra Rosenbaum, eds. *Fashion Prints in the Age of Louis XIV: Interpreting the Art of Elegance*. Lubbock: Texas Tech University Press and Los Angeles County Museum of Art, 2014, 8–14.

Teukolsky, Rachel (2009), *Victorian Writing and Modernist Aesthetics*, Oxford: Oxford University Press.

Theobald, J. (2004), *The Media and the Making of History*, Aldershot and Burlington: Ashgate Publishing.

Troy, N. (2003), *Couture Culture: A Study in Modern Art and Fashion*, Cambridge: MIT Press.

Vecellio, C. (1977), *Habiti Antichi et Moderni*, New York: Dover Publications.

von Boehn, M. (1966) *Puppen und Puppenspiele*. Josephine Nicoll (transl). New York.

Weller, S. (2007), "Fashion as Viscous Knowledge: Fashion's Role in Shaping Transnational Garment Production," *Journal of Economic Geography*, 7: 39–66.

Welters, L. and Abby Lillethun (2007), *The Fashion Reader*, Berg, Oxford.

Whiter, N. and J. Griffiths, eds. (2000), *The Fashion Business: Theory, Practice, Image*, Oxford: Berg.

Wilson, Sarah (2010), *The Visual World of French Theory: Figurations*, New Haven and London: Yale University Press.

Woozley, A. D. (1967), *Theory of Knowledge*, Hutchinson University Library, London.

INDEX